Prader-Willi Syndrome

Mary Lou Caldwell   Ronald L. Taylor
Editors

Prader-Willi Syndrome

Selected Research and Management Issues

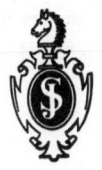

Springer-Verlag
New York Berlin Heidelberg
London Paris Tokyo

Mary Lou Caldwell
Ronald L. Taylor
Exceptional Student Education
Florida Atlantic University
Boca Raton, FL 33431-0991
USA

Library of Congress Cataloging-in-Publication Data
Prader-Willi syndrome.
   Bibliography: p.
   Includes indexes.
   1. Prader-Willi syndrome. I. Caldwell, Mary Lou.
II. Taylor, Ronald L., 1949–
RJ520.P7P74   1988   618.92′0043   87-37641

Typeset by Ampersand Publisher Services, Rutland, Vermont.

9 8 7 6 5 4 3 2 1

ISBN-13: 978-1-4612-8378-2   e-ISBN-13: 978-1-4612-3854-6
DOI:10.1007/13: 978-1-4612-3854-6

Preface

Prader-Willi syndrome was identified initially in 1956. The characteristics that were associated with Prader-Willi syndrome at that time were obesity, mental retardation, short stature, hypotonia in infancy, and cryptorchidism. Later, Prader and Willi added diminished fetal activity and a tendency to develop diabetes to the list of characteristics. Even today, diagnosis of Prader-Willi syndrome is made primarily on the basis of clinical phenotype.

As more and more individuals were diagnosed as having Prader-Willi syndrome, more attention was directed toward other characteristics (e.g., food-related behaviors) and management techniques, particularly related to weight control. The majority of information about Prader-Willi syndrome has come from case studies, parent reports, and other nonempirical sources. Until relatively recently, there was a paucity of empirical data-based studies investigating the diagnosis, characteristics, and management of individuals with Prader-Willi syndrome. Even today, research in this area is somewhat limited. Although much has been learned about this low incidence condition since 1956, there is still much more to learn. We are finding that some of the information about the syndrome has been supported by research, while other information has been questioned. New areas of research are investigating alternative and innovative methods of identification and treatment. Research related to the possible cytogenetic basis for the syndrome, differential diagnosis, unique characteristics of the syndrome, and the most effective management techniques has been conducted and should continue.

This book focuses on *selected* research and management issues related to Prader-Willi syndrome. It is not intended to be a comprehensive review of the syndrome, nor a "how to" book on treatment and management. In general, the book looks at the most recent advances in diagnosis, issues related to several nonmedical characteristics of the syndrome, recent research on a variety of management approaches, and the important area of parental concerns.

We would like to thank all of those who were instrumental in developing this book. Perhaps more importantly, we would like to thank those individuals with Prader-Willi syndrome with whom we have had the opportunity to work. Without them, the book would never have been conceived.

Contents

Contributors

Mary Lou Caldwell, PhD, Associate Professor, Exceptional Student Education, Florida Atlantic University, Boca Raton, Florida 33431-0991, USA

Suzanne B. Cassidy, MD, Associate Professor of Pediatrics, Director, Division of Human Genetics, University of Connecticut School of Medicine, Farmington, Connecticut 06032, USA

David H. Ledbetter, PhD, Associate Professor, Institute for Molecular Genetics, Baylor College of Medicine, Houston, Texas 77030, USA

James K. Luiselli, EdD, Clinical Psychologist, Behavioral and Educational Resource Associates, Concord, Massachusetts 01742, USA

Ronald L. Taylor, EdD, Professor, Exceptional Student Education, Florida Atlantic University, Boca Raton, Florida 33431-0991, USA

Charles W. Wagner, MD, Associate Professor, Surgery and Pediatrics, Arkansas Children's Hospital, University of Arkansas for Medical Sciences, Little Rock, Arkansas 72201, USA

1
Issues in Prader-Willi Syndrome: Diagnosis, Characteristics, and Management

JAMES K. LUISELLI, RONALD L. TAYLOR, and MARY LOU CALDWELL

Prader-Willi syndrome was described initially by Prader, Labhart, and Willi in a brief paper published in 1956. The characteristics comprising the syndrome included obesity, mental retardation, short stature, hypotonia in infancy, and cryptorchidism. The predominant behavioral features of the syndrome were hyperphagia and a compulsive preoccupation with food. In 1963, Prader and Willi supplemented their earlier work with a report on 14 additional cases. Added to the diagnostic picture were diminished fetal activity and a tendency to develop diabetes.

Beginning in the late 1960s, a series of publications appeared that confirmed other apparent cases of Prader-Willi syndrome while providing more detailed and extensive reviews of diagnostic criteria. Over the years, a relatively uniform clinical picture of Prader-Willi syndrome has emerged. The syndrome is characterized by a rather distinct combination of morphological and behavioral features and, in fact, diagnosis of the syndrome has been largely based on clinical phenotype. Only recently has progress been made in providing more laboratory-oriented data to establish a diagnosis (see Chapter 2).

The management of treatment of individuals with Prader-Willi syndrome has been of primary concern to parents and professionals alike. These treatment approaches have incorporated medical, educational, and behavioral techniques to provide a multidisciplinary management program. The techniques include surgery, pharmacological intervention, dietary management, and behavior modification. Much has been learned about the relative effectiveness of these and other therapeutic approaches for managing or modifying a variety of behaviors of this population.

This chapter provides a general introduction to the diagnosis, characteristics, and treatment of Prader-Willi syndrome. An overview of the syndrome will be presented through a description of its characteristics, followed by a discussion of the emergence and current status of therapeutic management approaches. Throughout the chapter, important research and management issues will be highlighted.

Diagnosis

Prader-Willi syndrome, like other syndromes, consists of a combination of physical and behavioral characteristics. Most of the work in the area of diagnosis has concentrated on identifying these characteristics and differentiating the syndrome from other congenital disorders. The following listing represents a compilation and description of diagnostic criteria. It should be noted that most of the early research regarding characteristics and behaviors were case studies, parent reports, and other nonempirical sources. Many of these characteristics/behaviors have been questioned and empirically investigated (see Chapter 3). Also, it is possible that because of our increased sophistication of diagnostic methods (see Chapter 2), many of the subjects described in the earlier studies would not be labeled as Prader-Willi syndrome. Conversely, it is possible that with our increased awareness of the syndrome, many individuals might now be labeled who before were misdiagnosed or not diagnosed at all.

WEIGHT

The weight of term newborn infants is often below normal and initial weight gain also may be very slow (Zellweger & Schneider, 1968). However, at around two years of age, weight increases and persistent appetite develops. This, in turn, leads to a condition of overweight such that most individuals with Prader-Willi syndrome become clinically obese.

HEIGHT

Height usually falls within normal limits during the first 10 years of life. An absence of prepubertal growth spurt is customary and by adulthood, height is usually under 5 feet (Homles et al., 1982).

CENTRAL NERVOUS SYSTEM AND INTELLECTUAL DEVELOPMENT

Infants typically are born following a normal, full-term pregnancy. Diminished fetal activity is frequently reported by the mother. Hypotonia is prevalent during infancy which deleteriously affects normal motor development. This condition results in the common description of a "floppy" baby. Sucking responses are also poor and this oral-motor dysfunction generally accounts for the slow weight gain normally observed during the first year of life (See Chapter 4 for a discussion of hypotonia and feeding problems). Most children with Prader-Willi syndrome learn to walk by 3 to 4 years of age, although their gait tends to be insecure. Delays in speech also are noted.

Intelligence quotients derived from standardized intelligence testing reportedly range from 20 to 90, with most falling within a 40 to 60 range (Zellweger & Schneider, 1968). Studying a sample of 32 persons with Prader-Willi syndrome, Hall and Smith (1972) reported a mean IQ score of 55 with a range of 18 to normal. Thus, utilizing AAMD classification criteria (American Association on Mental Deficiency, 1983), the majority of individuals afflicted with Prader-Willi syndrome are considered to be mildly to moderately mentally retarded. It is significant, of course, that some individuals test within normal limits. Chapter 3 addresses the issue of intellectual level and the pattern of cognitive deficits.

RESPIRATORY AND CARDIOPULMONARY FUNCTION

As a result of extreme obesity, some persons with Prader-Willi syndrome suffer from impaired breathing such that insufficient oxygen passes into the lungs. This so-called "Pickwickian syndrome" produces sleepiness, cyanosis, and potential heart failure. Deficient respiration also may result in an enlargement of the right side of the heart (cor pulmonale), described by some as the most common cause of death in Prader-Willi syndrome (Laurance, Brito, & Wilinson, 1981).

PSYCHOLOGICAL AND BEHAVIORAL FEATURES

The underlying condition of hyperphagia is associated with a number of behavioral problems that requires effective management. Food stealing and foraging are particularly prevalent disorders. Parents, for example, frequently report that their children are preoccupied with refrigerators and are constantly "scavenging" for food. It is also commonly reported that individuals with Prader-Willi syndrome search through trash containers, eat out of garbage pails, and consume unpalatable items such as frozen bread, animal food, and sticks of butter. Indiscriminate ingestion can lead to serious health problems, for example, intestinal obstruction or parasite infestations when nonfood products are consumed (pica). Johnston and Robertson (1977) reported the case of a 45-year-old woman with Prader-Willi syndrome who died from salt poisoning after consuming large quantities of jam topped with 3 to 4 tablespoons of salt. The behavioral management of a variety of eating-related behaviors is discussed in Chapter 5.

Persons with Prader-Willi syndrome are often described as being "manipulative," particularly surrounding efforts to acquire food. When denied access to consumable items through preventive measures (e.g., locked refrigerators), temper tantrums and acting-out behavior often may occur (Laurance et al., 1981). The prevalence of psychological/behavioral disturbance is underscored by Hall and Smith's (1972) estimate that some 70% of the persons diagnosed as having Prader-Willi syndrome display serious personality disorders. Chapter 3 includes information about the behavioral characteristics and Chapter 5 reviews the literature regarding the management of these behaviors.

FOOD PREFERENCES

It has been noted previously that a prevailing assumption in the understanding of Prader-Willi syndrome is that afflicted individuals possess indiscriminate food preferences. The generally accepted notion has been that quality of food is less important than quantity (Zellweger & Schneider, 1968). Until recently, however, empirical assessments of preferential eating by these individuals have not been conducted. Analyses of this type could affect the design of dietary regimens in several ways. For example, most programmed diets emphasize the provision of large quantities of low calorie (and perhaps nonpreferred) foods. If more preferred foods could be identified, then they could be included at smaller quantities with potentially fewer calories per mealtime serving; or preferred foods might be used to reinforce treatment progress (e.g., progressive weight loss) or alternative, adaptive behaviors.

Research by Caldwell and Taylor (Caldwell & Taylor, 1983; Taylor & Caldwell, 1986) has provided data related to food preferences in Prader-Willi syndrome. In these studies, individuals with the syndrome were given opportunities to select foods that varied in taste (sweet, salty, sour, plain). In the majority of cases, definite food preferences were revealed. When told they could consume smaller quantities of their preferred foods or larger quantities of their nonpreferred foods, nearly all subjects chose the lesser amount. Interestingly, one study (Caldwell & Taylor, 1983) found a relationship between cognitive functioning and food preferences. In it, individuals within a "nonretarded" group (average I.Q. = 77.7) demonstrated distinct preferences, whereas those in a "mildly retarded" group (average I.Q. = 62.8) did not. Since the majority of persons with Prader-Willi syndrome are classified as mildly to moderately retarded, this finding may account for the generally accepted assertion that within this population, food consumptioin is indiscriminate.

DIFFERENTIAL DIAGNOSIS

Prader-Willi is comprised of characteristics that overlap with other congenital disabilities. Accurate diagnosis is predicated on differentiating it from syndromes where commonalities are present.

Zellweger and Schneider (1968) distinguished two stages in Prader-Willi syndrome: (1) an infant hypotonic stage, and (2) a subsequent obesity stage. Hypotonia during infancy can occur in cases of cerebro-hepatorenal syndrome, Lowe's syndrome, neonatal myasthenia, and

Werdnig-Hoffman's disease (Holmes et al., 1972). For cerebrohepatorenal syndrome, differentiation from Prader-Willi syndrome is based upon the presence of craniofacial abnormalities and flexion contractures in the former condition. Lowe's syndrome is distinguished by the presence of cataracts, glaucoma, and aminoaciduria. Neonatal myasthenia can be identified on the basis of an edrophonium chloride test. Finally, electromyography and muscle biopsy can be utilized to differentiate Werdnig-Hoffman's disease.

Conditions of obesity, mental retardation, and hypogonadism in childhood are found in Laurence-Moon-Biedl syndrome, Frohlich's adiposogenital dystrophy, and Borjeson-Forssman-Lehmann syndrome. In Laurence-Moon-Biedl syndrome, other clinical features include retinitis pigmentosa and polydactyly. Children with adiposogenital dystrophy may not present with mental retardation, infant hypotonia, nor is hyperphagia a problem (Steffes, Holm, & Sulzbacher, 1981). Borjeson-Forssman-Lehmann syndrome is a rare disorder with an assumed X-linked, recessive gene transmission (Holmes et al., 1972).

Treatment

A variety of approaches have been attempted for the treatment of individuals with Prader-Willi syndrome. This section traces the evolution of intervention strategies and reviews the current status of therapeutic management and prevention. Since many of these topics are discussed at greater length in subsequent chapters, only a brief overview will be presented here.

ENVIRONMENTAL PREVENTION

The earliest assumptions regarding the treatment of individuals with Prader-Willi syndrome were that they evinced uncontrollable appetites and, as such, were unresponsive to only the most extreme methods of appetite management. Restrictive environmental arrangements such as bolted cabinets, locked refrigerators, and hidden food sources were commonly prescribed. Alterations of this type made it possible to prevent excessive pilfering of food but also were associated with an increase in behavioral difficulties, for example, temper tantrums, aggression, and the like. Also, such strategies, in and of themselves, did not lead to effective weight control. Although physically restricting access to food remains a component of most contemporary treatment plans, other intervention procedures must also be employed (Steffes et al., 1981).

SURGERY

Surgical interventions have been attempted for weight control with individuals with Prader-Willi syndrome but have met with limited success. Procedures such as gastric bypass, small intestinal bypass, and jaw wiring were reported in several publications (Bergsma, 1979; Soper, Mason, Printen, & Zellweger, 1975). These methods, of course, represent physically invasive procedures that, again, reflect the view that hunger is uncontrollable and must be managed through extreme means. Deleterious side effects also can occur with surgical procedures as in the cases of dehydration and liver damage following intestinal bypass (Bistrian, Blackburn, & Stanbury, 1977). Surgical approaches for a variety of problems are discussed in Chapter 6.

PHARMACOLOGY

Establishing control over hyperphagia has been attempted in some cases of Prader-Willi syndrome with the administration of appetite suppressing drugs such as dextroamphetamine (Zellweger, 1979). However, controlled clinical trials are lacking and, therefore, empirical support for this form of drug management awaits formal demonstration. A more recent pharmacological approach stems from the hypothesis that impaired appetite regulation in Prader-Willi syndrome may be a function of increased secretion of endogenous opiates in the brain (beta-endorphins). Administering Naloxone, an opiate antagonist, was demonstrated to be effective in decreasing food consumption in two persons with Prader-Willi syndrome (Kyriakides, Silverstone, Jeffcoate, & Laurance, 1980). Other reports describe a less successful outcome (Laurance et al., 1981) indicating that, to date, research findings must be regarded as equivocal.

DIET REGULATION

Beginning in the 1970s, a number of reports appeared focusing on the development of specially prescribed diets for use in a comprehensive treatment plan with individuals with Prader-Willi syndrome. Coplin, Hine, and Gormican (1976) employed a hypocaloric diet with eight children on an outpatient basis. After 6 months of dietary management, three of the eight children lost weight. Of note was the finding that as compared with a group of peers matched on age, height, and weight, the Prader-Willi sample required fewer calories to lose weight. In another study, Bistrian et al. (1977) treated four persons with Prader-Willi syndrome with a protein-sparing modified fast on an in-patient metabolic unit. Of the four individuals, only one was able to continue the diet and maintain weight loss as an out-patient.

Pipes and Holm (1973) described a weight control program for children with Prader-Willi syndrome that included individually designed diets for each child combined with adjunctive intervention strategies. In addition to the specialized diets, each child's nutrient intake, growth, and energy expenditure was carefully monitored coupled with adjustments in the diet regimens as age and stature changed. An essential ingredient in this program was the inclusion of parents and other natural change-agents (e.g., teachers) as integral members of a treatment team. In many ways, this program was a stepping stone for the evolution of broad-based management programs as we now know them, namely: (1) carefully formulated diets, (2) emphasis on out-patient treatment, (3) incorporation of paraprofessionals as interventionists, and (4) environmental prevention of food stealing and foraging.

BEHAVIORAL MANAGEMENT AND TRAINING

Another trend, originating about a decade ago, has been the application of behavior modification procedures both as a methodology to reduce management problems and increase adaptive responses. Most programs, for example, have incorporated some form of positive reinforcement to reward gradual reductions in weight, lowered caloric intake, and adherence to prescribed regimens. Various problem behaviors such as food stealing, tantrums, and aggression also have been treated successfully. One of the advantages of behavioral technology is that it can be imparted to natural change-agents such as parents and teachers. As a result, therapeutic intervention can be applied within multiple settings and extended on a 24 hour per day basis.

Steffes, Holm, & Sulzbacher (1981) have commented that, ideally, persons with Prader-Willi syndrome "should take responsibility for controlling their own obesity" (p. 8). Since the majority of these individuals are described as mildly to moderately retarded, they may possess the necessary cognitive and performance skills to self-manage some or all of their treatment plan. Self-management is a desirable clinical goal since it reduces the need for and time-demands required with externally imposed contingencies. Self-managed programs also can promote the long-term maintenance of therapy gains. Although few in number, programs employing self-control procedures in Prader-Willi syndrome have met with success (Altman, Bondy, & Hirsch, 1978) and are likely to be instituted with greater regularity in the coming years.

A final trend worth noting reflects the continued growth of behavioral medicine treatment and research. Behavioral medicine is the application of principles of learning to therapeutic management, risk reduction, and prevention of somatic disorders and medical problems. As related to Prader-Willi syndrome, methods can be utilized for such concerns as increasing energy expenditure through exercise, training nutritious food selection, and reducing stress associated with diagnostic and therapeutic medical procedures. Behavioral medicine applications in Prader-Willi syndrome should become more firmly established in the future as this discipline continues to evolve in the area of developmental disabilities (Luiselli, in press).

INCREASING ENERGY EXPENDITURE

The control and prevention of obesity is, for many, the primary goal of therapeutic management for individuals with Prader-Willi syndrome. Most obesity treatment specialists agree that potential reductions in fat composition and weight are not solely dependent on lowered caloric intake (Brownell, 1982). Rather, increasing energy expenditure in combination with dietary restrictions is considered to be the most advantageous weight management approach.

As mentioned in earlier sections, individuals with Prader-Willi syndrome are usually maintained on very restrictive, low-calorie diets (usually under 1,000 calories per day) to maintain their weight comparable with nonafflicted peers. Additional weight loss only follows further caloric reductions. The extremely low-calorie requirements in persons with the syndrome may be a function, in part, of diminished levels of physical activity. Children and young adults with Prader-Willi syndrome have been described as lethargic, sleepy, and easily fatigued (Hanson, 1981; Herrmann, 1981) as well as avoiding active physical play (Carman, 1981). However, empirical studies of activity levels and strategies to increase expenditure in Prader-Willi syndrome populations have only recently appeared.

Nardella, Sulzbacher, and Worthington-Roberts (1983) described a summer camp program for individuals with Prader-Willi syndrome in which physical activity was systematically monitored and reinforced. Twelve participants (ages 11 to 22 years) wore actometers and pedometers during a 2-week camp stay. Campers were provided a 1,000 calorie per day diet and regular exercise participation was scheduled and reinforced. As compared with a group of 13 similar-aged peers, the sample of Prader-Willi individuals displayed greater variability in daily exercise patterns. Weight losses of zero to 3.6 kg were obtained, with the greatest quantity of weight loss by those who were heaviest initially. Paradoxically, those individuals who lost the most weight were not the most physically active. As acknowledged by the authors, it may have been that the monitoring devices (particularly the actometer) measured motor responding that was not closely tied to the caloric expenditure required to affect weight loss.

In a study designed to increase activity levels, Caldwell, Taylor, and Bloom (1986) evaluated the effects of preferred (higher calorie) and nonpreferred (lower calorie) foods as reinforcement for exercise participation in a group of 11 individuals with Prader-Willi syndrome (average age = 21.5 years). The stimuli used as reinforcers were selected from a preferential tasting test. The reinforcers were selected for criterion performance on a variety of activities such as walking, swimming, cycling, and aerobic dancing. For 7 of the 11 participants, contingent reinforcement with preferred foods increased activity and exercise. This approach provides a relatively simple strategy to enhance caloric expenditure and is easily incorporated into applied settings.

INTERDISCIPLINARY MANAGEMENT

The multiplicity of intellectual, cognitive, and physical handicaps common to Prader-Willi syndrome demands a full spectrum of clinical services. History demonstrates that the earliest attempts at intervention concentrated on medical management, primarily to control obesity. Present-day approaches have subsequently evolved into a more interdisciplinary approach. As highlighted by Varni (1983), a distinction between *inter*disciplinary and *multi*disciplinary approaches should be considered:

Multidisciplinary refers to activities involving the efforts of professionals from a number of disciplines approaching the patient primarily through an uncoordinated discipline-specific fashion. This approach requires that each professional only know the skills specific to his/her own discipline. In contrast, the interdisciplinary approach requires that physicians, nurses, physical therapists, occupational therapists, medical social workers, psychologists, and other allied health professionals have a working knowledge of the other team members' skill and specialties. Thus, the interdisciplinary approach is synergistic, integrating the knowledge and skills from the various disciplines into a coordinated plan for patient care. (pp. 4–5)

Steffes et al. (1981) discussed the development of a clinic program at the University of Washington beginning in 1972. This clinic was the first devoted exclusively to the out-patient treatment of Prader-Willi syndrome. Professionals from the areas of medicine, psychology, nutrition, physical therapy, occupational therapy, speech and language pathology, and special education were united in a team-management format. Parent support services also were provided in an effort to alleviate the many stresses and difficulties confronting families of children with Prader-Willi syndrome.

Specialized programs like that developed at the University of Washington have begun at other university-affiliated clinics. It is clear that persons with Prader-Willi syndrome must be evaluated by multiple disciplines and that the resulting recommendations must be carried out in complementary fashion. Given the mandate of Public Law 94–142, children with Prader-Willi syndrome are entitled to specialized educational programming in the public schools. These children, therefore, most likely will remain in the home and, in effect, continue to place much of the burden of treatment on parents and other family members. Although the requirement of interdisciplinary management is acknowledged by parents and professionals alike, there remains the challenge of organizing and implementing clinic-based programs that efficiently combine diagnostic, treatment, evaluation, and outreach services. How we respond to this challenge will ultimately determine the future care of persons with Prader-Willi sydrome.

Summary

This chapter has served as an introduction to many research issues that focus on the diagnosis, characteristics, and treatment of Prader-Willi syndrome. Since its initial clinical description, much has been learned about the causes, sequelae, and management of this disability. More progress is needed, of course, in a variety of areas and, hopefully, with an eye towards prevention. Greater understanding and more effective treatment of Prader-Willi syndrome have evolved over the years thanks to many contributions from the areas of medicine, psychology, education, and rehabilitation. In the chapters that follow, several of these important issues are addressed. In Chapter 2, Ledbetter and Cassidy review the cytogenetic basis for Prader-Willi syndrome and report on the implications of new diagnostic techniques. In Chapter 3, Taylor discusses the areas of cognitive and behavioral characteristics associated with Prader-Willi syndrome and presents data that challenge some of the generally accepted views of those characteristics. In Chapter 4, Cassidy discusses the issues of hypotonia, developmental delay, and feeding problems that have implications for the management of infants with Prader-Willi syndrome. Luiselli reviews the behavioral literature associated with both Prader-Willi syndrome and the characteristics associated with the syndrome in Chapter 5. In Chapter 6, Wagner discusses surgical procedures that are available for individuals with Prader-Willi syndrome. Finally, Taylor and Caldwell address the important issue of parent concerns in Chapter 7 by reporting and summarizing data from a questionnaire.

REFERENCES

Altman, K., Bondy, A., & Hirsch, G. (1978). Behavioral tretment of obesity in patients with Prader-Willi syndrome. *Journal of Behavioral Medicine, 1,* 403–412.

American Association on Mental Deficiency. (1983). *Manual on terminology and classification in mental retardation.* Washington, DC: American Association on Mental Deficiency.

Bergsma, D. (Ed.). (1979). *Birth defects compendium.* New York: Liss.

Bistrian, B., Blackburn, G., & Stanbury, J. (1977). Metabolic aspects of a protein-sparing modified fast in the dietary management of Prader-Willi obesity. *New England Journal of Medicine, 295,* 774–779.

Brownell, K. D. (1982). Obesity: Understanding and treating a serious, prevalent, and refractory disorder. *Journal of Consulting and Clinical Psychology, 50,* 820–840.

Caldwell, M. L., & Taylor, R. L. (1983). A clinical note on food preference of individuals with Prader-Willi syndrome: The need for empirical research. *Journal of Mental Deficiency Research, 27,* 45–49.

Caldwell, M. L., Taylor, R. L., & Bloom, S. (1986). Use of preferential food as a reinforcer for increased activity of individuals with Prader-Willi syndrome. *Journal of Mental Deficiency Research, 30,* 347–354.

Carman, P. M. (1981). Physical exercise for children and adults with Prader-Willi syndrome. In V. A. Holm, S. Sulzbacher, & P. L. Pipes (Eds.), *The Prader-Willi syndrome.* Baltimore: University Park Press.

Coplin, S., Hine, J., & Gormican, A. (1976). Out-patient dietary management in the Prader-Willi syndrome. *Journal of the American Dietary Association, 68,* 330–334.

Hall, B. D., & Smith, D. W. (1972). Prader-Willi syndrome: A resume of 32 cases including an instance of affected first cousins, one of whom is of normal stature and intelligence. *Pediatrics, 81,* 286–293.

Hanson, J. W. (1981). A review of the etiology and pathogenesis of Prader-Willi syndrome. In V. A. Holm, S. Sulzbacher, & P. L. Pipes (Eds.), *The Prader-Willi syndrome.* Baltimore: University Park Press.

Herrmann, J. (1981). Implications of Prader-Willi syndrome for the individual and the family. In V. A. Holm, S. Sulzbacher, & P. L. Pipes (Eds.), *The Prader-Willi syndrome.* Baltimore: University Park Press.

Holmes, L. B., Moser, H. W., Halldorsson, S., Mack, C., Pant, S. S., & Matzilevich, B. (1972). *Mental retardation: An atlas of diseases with associated physical abnormalities.* New York: Macmillan.

Johnston, J. G., & Robertson, W. O. (1977). Fatal ingestion of table salt by an adult. *The Western Journal of Medicine, 126,* 141–143.

Kyriakides, M., Silverstone, T., Jeffcoate, W., & Laurance, B. (1980). Effect of naloxone on hyperphagia in Prader-Willi syndrome. *Lancet, 1,* 876–877.

Laurance, B. M., Brito, A., & Wilinson, J. (1981). Prader-Willi syndrome after age 15 years. *Archives of Disabilities in Childhood, 56,* 181–186.

Luiselli, J. K. (Ed.). (in press). *Behavorial medicine and development disabilities: An applied behavior analytic perspective.* New York: Springer-Verlag.

Nardella, M. T., Sulzbacher, S., & Worthington-Roberts, B. S. (1983). Activity levels of persons with Prader-Willi syndrome. *American Journal of Mental Deficiency, 87,* 498–505.

Pipes, P. L., & Holm V. A. (1973). Weight control of children with Prader-Willi syndrome. *Journal of the American Dietetic Association, 62,* 520–524.

Prader, A., Labhardt, A., & Willi, H. (1956). Ein syndrom von adipositas, kleinwuchs, kryptochismus and oligophrenie nach myatonieartigem zustand in neugeborenenalter. *Schweizerische Medizinische Wochenschrift, 86,* 1260–1261.

Soper, R. T., Mason, E. E., Printen, K. J., & Zellweger, H. (1975). Gastric bypass for morbid obesity in children and adolescents. *Journal of Pediatric Surgery, 10,* 51–58.

Steffes, M. J., Holm, V. A., & Sulzbacher, S. (1981). The Prader-Willi syndrome: Historical perspective. In V. A. Holm, S. Sulzbacher, & P. L. Pipes (Eds.), *The Prader-Willi syndrome.* Baltimore: University Park Press.

Taylor, R. L., & Caldwell, M. L. (1986). Type and strength of food preferences of individuals with Prader-Willi syndrome. *Journal of Mental Deficiency Research, 30,* 181–185.

Varni, J. W. (1983). *Clinical behavioral pediatrics.* New York: Pergamon.

Zellweger, H. (1979). Prader-Willi syndrome. In D. Bergsma (Ed.), *Birth defects compendium.* New York: Liss.

Zellweger, H., & Schneider, H. J. (1968). Syndrome of hypotonia-hypomentia-obesity (HHHO) or Prader-Willi syndrome. *American Journal of Diseases of Children, 115,* 588–598.

2
The Etiology of Prader-Willi Syndrome: Clinical Implications of the Chromosome 15 Abnormalities

DAVID H. LEDBETTER AND SUZANNE B. CASSIDY

The etiology and pathogenesis of the Prader-Willi syndrome have been focuses of interest and conjecture since the first description of the disorder by Prader, Labhart, and Willi (1956). Until recently, clinical investigations failed to demonstrate any consistent anatomical, biochemical, chromosomal, or structural abnormality that would explain the multiple manifestations of this condition or could be used to confirm a clinical diagnosis. In fact, in the vast majority of cases, the condition is still diagnosed on the basis of characteristic clinical features and natural history. Only since 1981 have we been able to confirm the clinical impression of Prader-Willi syndrome through cytogenetic analysis in the majority of cases (Ledbetter, Riccardi, Airhart, Strobel, Keenan, & Crawford, 1981; Ledbetter, Mascarello, Riccardi, Harper, Airhart, & Strobel, 1982). The etiology in the remaining cases is still unclear.

Prior to 1981, attempts to understand the cause of Prader-Willi syndrome were largely based upon observation and deduction. Clarren and Smith (1977) noted the abnormalities of morphogenesis, growth, and function in the syndrome and postulated that a disturbance in the development and function of midline structures of the brain, including thalamus and hypothalamus, could result in the majority of manifestations that are characteristic of this disorder. They suggested that a single localized defect in early brain development could cause: (1) hypotonia; (2) hypothalamic dysfunctions leading to growth abnormalities, hypogonadism, and abnormal appetite control; (3) small frontal brain leading to cognitive dysfunction, a narrow bifrontal diameter, and upslanting palpebral fissures. This postulated cause of Prader-Willi syndrome was reiterated by Hanson (1981), who suggested the possibility of etiologic heterogeneity since a number of disturbances could be envisioned as resulting in a localized midline brain defect and consequently the features noted in Prader-Willi syndrome. The few postmortem neuropathologic studies of individuals with Prader-Willi syndrome, however, fail to demonstrate a gross or microscopic defect of any portion of the brain, including the midline structures (Bray, Dahms, Swerdloff, Fiser, Atkinson,

& Carrel, 1983; Laurance, Brito, & Wilkinson, 1981; Zellweger & Schneider, 1968).

Cytogenetic Basis for Prader-Willi Syndrome

EARLY STUDIES BY ROUTINE METHODS

The first suggestion that Prader-Willi syndrome might be associated with a specific chromosome as part of its etiology came from Hawkey and Smithies (1976) who reported a patient with a balanced translocation involving both members of the number 15 chromosome pair. Their review of the literature showed 10 cases of chromosome abnormalities in 61 patients previously studied, with 3 of these 10 involving a D group chromosome (numbers 13, 14, or 15). Since these studies were conducted prior to chromosome banding techniques, the individual D group chromosome could not be identified, but Hawkey and Smithies commented that "it would be tempting to speculate that the number 15 chromosome is involved in its (Prader-Willi syndrome) pathogenesis." This speculation was supported by the publication of seven additional cases of translocations involving chromosome 15 over the next 3 years (reviewed in Ledbetter et al., 1981). Several authors suggested that since loss of material on the short arm of chromosome 15 was a common denominator in all translocations, this was the etiologically important event and accounted for 10 to 15% of all Prader-Willi syndrome cases. Subsequently, it was shown by high-resolution chromosome techniques that subtle chromosome 15 abnormalities involving the long arm, not observable by routine methods, account for the *majority* of cases (Ledbetter et al., 1981; 1982).

HIGH-RESOLUTION CHROMOSOME ANALYSIS

What is meant by the term high-resolution chromosome analysis? The number of bands seen along the length of a chromosome is not constant, but is a function of the stage of the cell cycle. Chromosomes go through an extreme process of contraction from a highly dispersed interphase appearance to a highly contracted state at late metaphase. Each chromosome band seen in metaphase is actually comprised of 2 to 4 bands observable in the earlier stage of prometaphase. Since a much larger number of bands is present at prometaphase, detection of smaller deletions or duplications is possible.

Routine chromosome techniques involve a relatively long treatment (20 minutes to 1 hour or longer) with agents that arrest cells in mitosis, such as colchicine, to accumulate a small proportion of dividing cells from an asynchronous cell population. Most of these cells will be arrested in mid- to late metaphase, when an average chromosome has less than 20 distinct bands along its length and the total haploid set of 23 chromosomes has about 300 to 400 bands. A very small proportion of cells will be in the earlier stage of prometaphase, which has approximately 550 to 850 bands. It is possible, however, to enrich the percentage of cells in earlier stages of mitosis by cell synchronization techniques (e.g., Yunis, 1976).

The technical process of synchronizing lymphocyte cultures requires additional handling and expense, but the more important difficulty in high-resolution cytogenetics is the microscopic analysis of these more elongated chromosomes. Although more potential information is present, the degree of difficulty identifying each chromosome and region of a chromosome is correspondingly higher. Therefore only the most experienced technicians in a lab are usually able to perform this type of analysis, and not all cytogenetic laboratories offer high-resolution studies. Because of the additional time and expense involved in these analyses, it is impossible to apply them to all routine cytogenetic referrals, although they are essential to detect certain subtle deletions.

SMALL DELETION OF 15q DISCOVERED BY HIGH RESOLUTION TECHNIQUES

Because of the cases of chromosome 15 involvement, Ledbetter et al. (1981;1982) applied high-resolution methods to patients with Prader-Willi syndrome. A small, interstitial deletion in the proximal portion of the long arm of chromosome 15 (see Figure 2.1) was observed in more than 50% of the patients studied. The chromosome band missing in these patients, designated q12, cannot be seen in most routine cytogenetic preparations and, in fact, many of the patients with deletions had been studied previously by routine methods and found to have normal karyotypes.

Thus it was not until 1982 that it was demonstrated that the majority of patients with Prader-Willi syndrome had a specific cytogenetic abnormality. It is important to remember that any normal chromosome result on an individual with Prader-Willi syndrome obtained prior to 1981 to 1982 refers to a routine cytogenetic study and should be repeated with high-resolution techniques. After this time, experienced labs should have performed high-resolution studies with specific attention to ruling out a small deletion in 15q. In the case of studies of individuals with Prader-Willi syndrome, the written report from the lab should indicate whether routine or high-resolution studies (alternatively called prophase, prometaphase, or elongated chromosome studies) were performed. Specific mention of attention to chromosome 15 should also be included, and whether the interstitial deletion was present or absent.

At least nine surveys examining 195 patients with Prader-Willi syndrome using high-resolution cytogenetic techniques have now been repor-

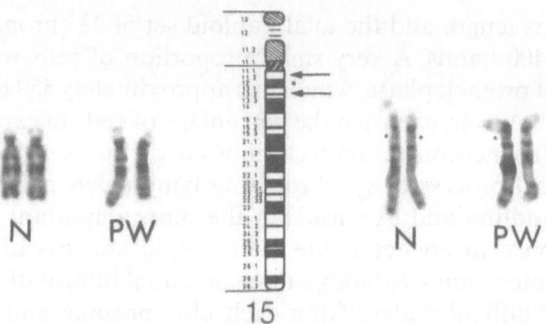

FIGURE 2.1. Idiogrammatic representation and G-banded photographs of chromosome 15 from normal and Prader-Willi syndrome individuals. In the center is an idiogram of chromosome 15 at the 850-band stage of prometaphase. The critical region deleted in Prader-Willi syndrome is the q11-q12 segment (the q12 band is indicated by a dot and the presumed breakpoints by arrows). To the left are G-banded photographs of the chromosome 15 pair from a normal individual and a patient with Prader-Willi syndrome at about the 400-band stage (midmetaphase) obtained by routine chromosome techniques. The q11-q12 bands are not discernible, and it is difficult to tell the difference between the patient and the normal individual. On the right are G-banded photographs of the chromosome 15 pair from a normal subject and an individual with Prader-Willi syndrome at approximately the 850-band stage (prometaphase). Note the presence of the q11-q12 bands in both homologs in the normal individual, but only the homolog on the left in the individual with Prader-Willi syndrome, indicating a deletion in the homolog on the right (q12 band indicated by a dot).

ted (see Table 2.1). The frequency of chromosome 15 abnormalities detected varies from just over 50 to 100% in these surveys. The most common finding is a small interstitial deletion (60%), although other anomalies of chromosome 15 have been reported.

Most Deletions Are De Novo

In six of the nine surveys, parental chromosome studies were done in some of the deletion cases. Most parental studies have been normal, indicating that the deletions are usually de novo events (i.e., new mutations). However, a relatively small number of cases have been studied, and we cannot rule out the theoretical possibility of a balanced insertional translocation in a parent as has been seen in both the aniridia-Wilms tumor deletion of chromosome 11 (Hittner, Riccardi, & Francke, 1979; Kousseff & Agatucci, 1981; Yunis and Ramsay, 1980) and the retinoblastoma deletion of chromosome 13 (Rivera, Turleau, de Grouchy, Junien, Despoisse & Zucker, 1981; Strong, Riccardi, Ferrell & Sparkes, 1981). Two cases from the high-resolution surveys of Prader-Willi syndrome are possible exam-

TABLE 2.1. High-resolution cytogenetic surveys of Prader-Willi syndrome.

	Ledbetter et al. (1981, 1982)	Mattei et al. (1983)	Cassidy et al. (1984)	Fukushima et al. (1984)[a]	Fear et al. (1985)	Niikawa & Ishikiriyama (1985)	Labidi & Cassidy (1986)	Butler et al. (1986)	Takano et al. (1986)	Total
Deletion (15)	23	8	11[b]	11	6	15	9	21	12	116 (59.5%)
Other 15 abnormality	2[c]	1[d]	1[e]		1[f]	2[g]				7 (3.6%)
Normal	20	8		1	5	10	4	18	6	72 (37.0%)
Total	45	17	12	12	12	27	13	39	18	195
Phenotypic difference Deletion vs. normal	Y	Y	N	N	N	Y	N	Y	N	

Note. Y = yes; N = no.
[a]Excludes patients also described in Niikawa & Ishikiriyama (1985). [b]Includes 2 mosaic deletion cases. [c]1 case: 45,XY,rob(15;15)(p11;p11); 1 case: 46,XX/47,XX,+idic(15)(q11). [d]47,XY,+idic(15)(q11). [e]45,XY,−7,−15,+der(7),t(7;15)(q36;q13). [f]46,XY,−15,−22,+der(22),t(15;22)(q13;q11.2)pat. [g]2 cases: 45,t(15;15)(p11;q12-q13).

ples of such a balanced insertional event. Fear, Mutton, Berry, Heckmatt, & Dubowitz (1985) described a smaller than usual deletion in one patient with Prader-Willi syndrome and the same deletion in the normal father. They suggested this may represent a normal variant, but a balanced translocation was not considered or ruled out. Niikawa and Ishikiriyama (1985) found a deletion in the normal mother of one patient. They looked for, but could not find, evidence of an insertional translocation event. Thus, parental balanced insertional translocations in Prader-Willi syndrome remain a theoretical concern, but no documented case has yet been described. Given that the overall recurrence risk for Prader-Willi syndrome is less than 1%, it may be difficult to justify the cost of high-resolution cytogenetic studies on all parents of deletion cases.

Parental Origin of De Novo Deletions

Chromosomal polymorphism studies have been performed on the normal parents of deletion cases to determine the parental origin of the deleted chromosome. In one series, 13 of 13 cases were paternal in origin (Butler, Meaney, & Palmer, 1986). In a second series, six of seven cases were paternal (Niikawa & Ishikiriyama, 1985). These findings are consistent with a previous study demonstrating preferential paternal origin of various de novo structural chromosome rearrangements (Chamberlin & Magenis, 1980). Thus, unlike nondisjunction events producing trisomy that preferentially occur in female meiosis, structural chromosome abnormalities seem to be more common in male meiosis. Epidemiologic studies of fathers of de novo deletion cases may be useful in identifying factors that affect spermatogenesis and predispose to chromosomal rearrangements.

Population Frequency of 15q Deletion

Accurate information regarding the frequency of Prader-Willi syndrome is lacking, but a reasonable estimate is 1:10,000 births (Holm, 1981). Since the 15q deletion occurs in at least 50% of these individuals, the frequency of the deletion would be 1:20,000 or greater. The most common chromosome deletion is generally considered to be the deletion of the short arm of chromosome 5 in the cri du chat syndrome, with a frequency estimated at 1:50,000 births (Niebuhr, 1978). Therefore, the *15q deletion of Prader-Willi syndrome is probably the most common chromosomal deletion in man,* and may be more than twice as frequent as the next most common deletion, 5p.

NORMAL CHROMOSOMES—IS IT PRADER-WILLI SYNDROME?

The second most common finding in the cytogenetics surveys of Prader-Willi syndrome is a normal karyotype. Thirty-seven percent of the 195 individuals studied had normal karyotypes (see Table 2.1). This frequency varies from 0 to 47% and may be influenced by clinical criteria for inclusion in the study. According to Holm (1981), the diagnosis of the syndrome is dependent on the presence of all of the following cardinal features: hypotonia, hypogonadism, obesity, short stature, dysmorphic facial features, and dysfunctional central nervous system performance. Most studies with a high rate of chromosomally normal results note that the normal karyotype group is clinically more heterogeneous than the deletion group and includes patients having atypical features or lacking one or more of the essential features. Studies with lower frequencies of normal chromosome results tended to use more strict inclusion criteria for Prader-Willi syndrome and therefore saw no clinical difference between normal karyotype and deletion cases. This trend suggests that when only typical patients with Prader-Willi syndrome are considered, 70 to 90% will demonstrate chromosome 15 abnormalities. This still leaves 10 to 30% of patients with all classical features of the syndrome but no visible chromosome abnormality. A submicroscopic deletion or other alteration on chromosome 15 is possible, and this may be clarified by future molecular studies. Obviously, in the case of normal chromosomes, parental studies are unnecessary.

TRANSLOCATIONS

Of 123 cases of Prader-Willi syndrome with chromosome abnormalities, five (4%) had translocations involving chromosome 15. Recent literature reviews have documented at least 30 cases of chromosome 15 translocations in Prader-Willi syndrome (Charrow, Balkin, & Cohen, 1983; Duckett, Roberts, & Davies, 1984; Mattei, Souiah & Mattei, 1984), but this larger number reflects a bias of ascertainment due to the ability to detect gross chromosomal rearrangements prior to 1981 using routine cytogenetic methods. The translocations are usually unbalanced, producing monosomy for the same proximal long arm region of 15 as is found in interstitial deletions. However, many cases are apparently balanced translocations, suggesting disruption of a single genetic locus or a position effect (Lejeune, Maunoury, Prieur, & van den Akker, 1979).

Parental studies are particularly important in translocation cases. Six of 30 (20%) cases in the literature involve familial rearrangements, which may significantly increase recurrence risk. To date, only one familial recurrence of Prader-Willi syndrome has been reported due to a familial balanced translocation (Hasegawa, et al., 1984). Unfortunately, in some of the balanced translocation cases, normal family members carry the same rearrangement as the Prader-Willi syndrome proband (Berry, Wittingham, & Neville, 1981; Smith & Noel, 1980; Wu, Hasen, & Warburton, 1981), making counseling issues related to diagnosis and prognosis extremely difficult.

ADDITIONAL MARKER CHROMOSOMES

Two cases (1.6%) in Table 2.1 and additional cases in the literature (reviewed by Mattei et al., 1984) describe Prader-Willi syndrome associated with an extra marker chromosome derived from chromosome 15. This is a unique circumstance in human cytogenetics in which trisomy (three copies) or tetrasomy (four copies) of a specific chromosome region causes the same phenotype as monosomy (one copy). We currently have no reasonable explanation for how this might occur. All cases so far have been de novo, so that recurrence risk is minimal.

CHROMOSOME 15 ABNORMALITIES—CAUSE OR EFFECT OF PRADER-WILLI SYNDROME?

This variety of abnormalities affecting a single region of chromosome 15 has led to some controversy in the literature as to whether or not the cytogenetic abnormalities are the cause of the syndrome as originally suggested (Ledbetter et al., 1981; 1982) or one of the effects of some other etiologic factor (Kousseff, 1982). As a laboratory diagnostic tool it really doesn't matter whether the chromosome 15 abnormality is cause or effect. However, it is our opinion that the chromosome 15 abnormalities are most likely the primary cause of the majority of cases for the following reasons:

1. The great majority (>95%) of the abnormalities produce a consistent genetic effect, that is, monosomy for the segment 15q11-q13. The apparently balanced, trisomic, or tetrasomic cases are rare (<5%).
2. If chromosome 15 lability were an effect of Prader-Willi syndrome, the rearrangements would all be postzygotic events. This would predict a high frequency of mosaicism, that is, mixtures of normal cell lines with abnormal cell lines and even multiple different chromosome 15 abnormalities within the same patient. It would also predict that both 15 homologs might frequently be involved, which is not the case.

Clearly, there is much left to be learned about the association of chromosome 15 abnormalities and Prader-Willi syndrome. We don't know whether there is one or many genes on chromosome 15 whose abnormal genetic dosage produces the Prader-Willi syndrome phenotype. (This is, of course, also true of all cytogenetic disorders). Isolation and characterization of DNA probes that fall within the critical region on chromosome 15 should go a long way in improving our understanding of this unusual genetic disorder. Fortunately, our lack of understanding of how cytogenetic imbalances produce a specific clinical disorder does not decrease their practical usefulness.

Clinical Implications of Cytogenetic Findings

THE VALUE OF CYTOGENETIC FINDINGS

Since not every person with the clinical features of Prader-Willi syndrome has a 15q deletion, and since the vast majority of cases are sporadic with very little chance for subsequent children to be affected, there is a logical question related to the purpose of performing a prometaphase chromosome analysis in a patient suspected of having the syndrome. In which clinical situation should the study be conducted? At what point in the life of the individual should the study be conducted? How can individuals and families benefit from the results, both positive (del 15q) and negative (normal)? These are important and frequently asked questions, and are sometimes difficult to answer.

In the infant who is hypotonic without apparent cause, multiple expensive and invasive tests are frequently performed to find the cause of the hypotonia. Prader-Willi syndrome is one of the more common causes (Berry et al., 1981). If prometaphase chromosome analyses were performed in all infants with hypotonia of unknown cause, particularly those in whom cryptorchidism or genital hypoplasia is a feature, the majority of people with Prader-Willi syndrome would be recognized in the first few months of life. The benefits of early diagnosis are many, including: (1) reassurance that the hypotonia will improve and become minimally significant, (2) assurance that efforts to compensate for feeding problems will be successful and such problems will resolve, (3) avoidance of invasive and expensive testing such as muscle biopsy, (4) an indication for early involvement in physical therapy to avoid the complications of infantile hypotonia (see Chapter 4, this volume), (5) the psychological benefits to the family of having a specific diagnosis and relatively predictable outcome, and (6) the knowledge that recurrence risk is very low, which may be important for family planning purposes. While the diagnosis is not ruled out by the absence of a 15q deletion, the potential benefits when a deletion is found seem to justify the expense.

In the developmentally delayed toddler or young child with features suggestive of Prader-Willi syndrome, the performance of a prometaphase chromosome analysis may help to end the search for a diagnosis. The knowledge that there is a specific and real cause for developmental problems, or the confirmation of a suspected clinical diagnosis, often has a tremendous psychological benefit for parents. Many parents were considered "bad parents" because their child was not doing what he or she should do developmentally, and many wrongly blame themselves for the delay. The establishment of a diagnosis with a positive cytogenetic finding also has the benefit of helping to assure appropriate programming in the school system. In addition, parents of developmentally delayed children will often decide to avoid having more children until they know the prognosis for the delayed child and the recurrence risk for subsequent children. The finding of a 15q deletion provides a specific diagnosis, information about natural history of the disorder, the specific areas in which intervention is needed, and knowledge that the recurrence risk is minimal.

In the older child or adult who manifests many features of Prader-Willi syndrome, there are additional benefits of chromosome analysis. Lack of secondary sex characteristics and primary amenorrhea are major features of the disorder, and extensive evaluations are often done in search of a cause. Confirmation of the diagnosis with the finding of a 15q deletion can avoid that search. In addition, siblings of adults with intellectual handicaps often are concerned about their risks of having affected offspring. The finding of a 15q deletion helps to reassure them of a negligible risk.

It should be remembered, however, that the absence of the 15q deletion does not preclude the possibility of Prader-Willi syndrome. In the small percentage of cases in which a chromosomal translocation or unusual chromosome arrangement involving chromosome 15 is found to be the cause of the Prader-Willi syndrome phenotype, recurrence risks may be increased, and family studies may be necessary. Alternatively, a different chromosome defect may be found to be the cause of the features which led to consideration of the diagnosis of Prader-Willi syndrome and such a finding would also be of benefit in understanding prognosis and recurrence risks. For all these reasons, it is of value to obtain prometaphase cytogenetic analysis when the diagnosis of Prader-Willi syndrome is considered.

EARLY DIAGNOSIS AND PROGNOSIS

The discovery of the 15q deletion in Prader-Willi syndrome is a new one, and no cases of the syndrome diagnosed at birth and followed long-term are available. Nonetheless, it is the anecdotal impression of those taking care of large numbers of people with this disorder that the prognosis is improved by early diagnosis and intervention. The many advantages of early diagnosis are mentioned above in discussing the value of cytogenetic analysis in the hypotonic infant. When the diagnosis is made only after obesity has set in, the weight management problem in Prader-Willi syndrome is more difficult to handle, and poor eating habits must be corrected rather than merely avoided. The value of early intervention and infant stimulation has been demonstrated in other disorders, and should apply equally to Prader-Willi syndrome. Entry into such programs often awaits a diagnosis, thus losing valuable time. Educational programming also can be improved by being responsive to their known cognitive strengths and weaknesses. The psychological adaptation of a family to a developmentally delayed child also has been demonstrated to be improved when a cause for the problems is identified, and the diminution of interparental conflict and its consequent high rate of broken families is a further benefit of early diagnosis.

WHERE TO OBTAIN HIGH-RESOLUTION CYTOGENETIC STUDIES FOR PRADER-WILLI SYNDROME

As mentioned previously, high-resolution chromosome analysis is difficult and time-consuming. Although most laboratories will offer high-resolution on a service basis (sometimes at a higher charge than routine studies), the amount of experience a lab has with Prader-Willi syndrome diagnosis will be quite variable. It is our personal experience that the subtle deletion in chromosome 15 associated with Prader-Willi syndrome is the *single most difficult cytogenetic diagnosis to make accurately*. Since the number of cases that any one lab would handle is relatively small, this is perhaps the best example of a cytogenetic disorder where referral of specimens to more experienced reference laboratories should be considered. To determine this, one should consult with a genetics counselor, medical geneticist, or directly with the cytogenetics lab director. They will be able to determine whether they are experienced and comfortable with the diagnosis of Prader-Willi syndrome, prefer to refer the specimen elsewhere, or perhaps perform the studies in parallel with another laboratory.

FAMILIAL IMPLICATIONS AND GENETIC COUNSELING

When a 15q deletion has been identified in an individual clinically suspected of having Prader-Willi syndrome, it is possible to provide the parents with specific information and options. First, as mentioned above, several studies have shown that such deletions are most often de novo. Based upon our current knowledge, we can therefore reassure such families that there was nothing that either parent did or did not do, prior to or during the pregnancy, that is known to have caused or predisposed to this chromosome anomaly. Next, we can state that the parents are not at substantially greater risk of having subsequent children with Prader-Willi syndrome than is anyone in the general population. Finally, we can likewise assure the parents that their other children are not at increased risk of having similarly affected children. The issue of recurrence risk in the offspring of people who themselves have Prader-Willi syndrome with a 15q deletion is unclear, but since the profound hypogonadism associated with the syndrome causes infertility, this is not a real issue.

When the 15q deletion is not present in a person suspected of having Prader-Willi syndrome, the situation is considerably less clear. It is known that a minority of people with the characteristic clinical features of the syndrome do not have this cytogenetic anomaly, and that most of them appear to be no different clinically from those who do. Whether the cause of the syndrome in these cases is the same or different will have to await further progress in the molecular studies of DNA probes in the critical region of the 15q deletion. Nonetheless, only a very small number of couples have had more than one affected child with Prader-Willi syndrome, and there is probably less than a 0.1% chance that an individual who has a chromosomally normal child with the syndrome will have another affected child (Cassidy, 1987). It is only when there is an unusual cytogenetic anomaly such as a chromosome translocation as the basis for Prader-Willi syndrome that an increased recurrence risk can be quoted with some degree of certainty. Such cases should be handled with the consultation of a geneticist.

PRENATAL DIAGNOSIS

Unfortunately, it is very difficult to routinely achieve a 550 to 850 band resolution from either chorion villus cells or amniotic fluid cells. The synchronization methods that work well for lymphocyte cultures do not work as well for other cell types. In any individual case, a small percentage of sufficiently long chromosomes in prometaphase may be found to make the diagnosis, but this is variable and too unpredictable to offer as a routine clinical service. Until better techniques are developed, we agree with Schinzel (1986) that is is unreasonable to put the diagnostic laboratory in the position of trying to make this cytogenetic diagnosis with amniotic fluid or chorion villus cells. Routine prenatal chromosome studies could be offered to rule out other common abnormalities (e.g., trisomies) on the basis of the high anxiety of parents with one handicapped child due to a chromosome abnormality. Schinzel (1986) also has suggested that ultrasound monitoring of fetal movement may aid in prenatal diagnosis, although to our knowledge this approach has not been attempted.

The chromosome resolution would be much greater from a fetal blood specimen, but sampling procedures for fetal blood are available at relatively few centers. Sampling by fetoscopy is associated with a 4 to 5% risk of fetal loss (International Fetoscopy Group, 1984), significantly greater than that of amniocentesis. Although complete data are not yet available, the newer method of fetal blood sampling by direct ultrasound guidance appears to have a much lower risk than fetoscopy (Daffos, Capella-Pavlovsky, & Forestier, 1983; Hobbins, Grannum, Romero, Reece, & Mahoney, 1985), and could make prenatal high-resolution chromosome studies possible. Development of molecular probes specific to this region of 15 may someday provide a more straightforward method of prenatal diagnosis of Prader-Willi syndrome utilizing chorion villus or amniotic fluid cells.

In the case of de novo translocations or extra markers, recurrence risk is extremely low. However, unlike deletion cases, detection of the translocation or marker is relatively easy using either chorion villus or amniotic fluid cells and could be considered. Obviously, for familial translocation cases, prenatal diagnosis is strongly advised.

Future Research Directions

A better understanding of the relationship between the chromosome 15 abnormalities and Prader-Willi syndrome will most likely come from research aimed at characterization of this chromosomal region at a molecular level. Donlon, Lalande, Wyman, Bruns, & Latt (1986) have successfully constructed an enriched chromosomal library for the proximal long arm of chromosome 15, which has allowed them to identify DNA probes that are deleted in patients with Prader-Willi syndrome with visible cytogenetic deletions. Additional probes need to be isolated, characterized, and tested against a large number of patients with the syndrome. The goals of this type of research are several fold: (1) Probes may be identified that allow detection of a deletion on a molecular level when no cytogenetic deletion is visible, thus increasing the sensitivity of our diagnostic capabilities. With such probes, a deletion might be detected in all patients with the syndrome; (2) Diagnosis of deletions with molecular techniques may eventually become simpler than the technically difficult method of high-resolution cytogenetics, and may be applicable to prenatal diagnostic situations where chromosome detection is currently not feasible; (3) Molecular characterization may provide insight into the cause of the extreme lability of this region as reflected in the numerous chromosome rearrangements, and may aid our understanding of causes of structural chromosome rearrangements that occur in spermatogenesis; (4) Molecular characterization will eventually provide us information on the nature of the genes that are located within the critical region and perhaps provide insight into their role in the pathogenesis of Prader-Willi syndrome.

Summary

The establishment of a cytogenetic abnormality involving chromosome 15 as the cause of the Prader-Willi syndrome is a relatively recent event with important clinical and practical implications. Detection of this subtle abnormality (usually a deletion) requires sophisticated high-resolution cytogenetic techniques not available in all laboratories. A minority of patients with the syndrome show no visible deletion, suggesting that submicroscopic deletions may occur or that other etiologies produce the same phenotype. Therefore, detection of a chromosome 15 abnormality is strong confirmation of the diagnosis, but normal chromosome results do not rule it out. Detection of the deletion in a newborn or young child not only establishes a diagnosis, but also allows early intervention in th. ireas of weight management and educatioinal planning. Since the chromosome abnormalities are virtually all de novo events, families can be reassured of an extremely low recurrence risk (<0.1%) for the disorder. Although there is still much to be learned about the cause of this frequent chromosome abnormality and how it produces the features of Prader-Willi syndrome, many practical benefits are already apparent from our new ability to detect a specific chromosomal basis for this unique disorder.

REFERENCES

Berry, A. C., Wittingham, A. G., & Neville, B. G. R. (1981). Chromosome 15 in floppy infants. *Archives of Disease in Childhood, 56,* 882–885.

Bray, G. A., Dahms, W. T., Swerdloff, R. S., Fiser, R. H., Atkinson, R. L., & Carrel, R. E. (1983). The Prader-Willi syndrome: A study of 40 patients and a review of the literature. *Medicine, 62,* 59–80.

Butler, M. G., Meaney, F. J., & Palmer, C. G. (1986). Clinical and cytogenetic survey of 39 individuals with Prader-Labhart-Willi syndrome. *American Journal of Medical Genetics, 23,* 793–809.

Cassidy, S. B., Thuline, H. C., & Holm, V. A. (1984). Deletion of chromosome 15(q11-13) in a Prader-Labhart-Willi syndrome clinic population. *American Journal of Medical Genetics, 17,* 485–495.

Cassidy, S. B. (1987). Letter to the Editor: Recurrence risk in Prader-Willi syndrome. *American Journal of Medical Genetics, 28,* 59–60.

Chamberlin, J., & Magenis, R. E. (1980). Parental origin of de novo chromosome rearrangements. *Human Genetics 53,* 343–347.

Charrow, J., Balkin, N., & Cohen, M. M. (1983). Translocations in Prader-Willi syndrome. *Clinical Genetics, 23,* 304–307.

Clarren, S. K., & Smith, D. W. (1977). Prader-Willi syndrome: Variable severity and recurrence risk. *American Journal of Diseases of Children, 131,* 789–800.

Daffos, F., Capella-Pavolvsky, M., & Forestier, F. (1983). Fetal blood sampling via the umbilical cord using a needle guided by ultrasound: Report of 66 cases. *Prenatal Diagnosis, 3,* 271–277.

Donlon, T. A., Lalande, M., Wyman, A., Bruns, G., & Latt, S. A. (1986). Isolation of molecular probes associated with the chromosome 15 instability in the Prader-Willi syndrome. *Proceedings of the National Academy of Sciences (USA), 83,* 4408–4412.

Duckett, D. P., Roberts, S. H., & Davies, P. (1984). Unbalanced reciprocal translocations in cases of Prader-Willi syndrome. *Human Genetics, 67,* 156–161.

Fear, C. N., Mutton, D. E., Berry, A. C., Heckmatt, J. Z., & Dubowitz, V. (1985). Chromosome 15 in Prader-Willi syndrome. *Developmental Medicine and Child Neurology, 27,* 305–311.

Fukushima, Y., Niikawa, N., & Kuroki, Y. (1984). The Prader-Willi syndrome and interstitial deletion of chromosome 15: High-resolution chromosome analyses of 14 patients with the Prader-Willi syndrome and of 5 suspected infants. *Japanese Journal of Human Genetics, 29,* 1–6.

Hanson, J. W. (1981). A view of the etiology and pathogenesis of Prader-Willi syndrome. In V. A. Holm, S. Sulzbacher, & P. L. Pipes (Eds.), *Prader-Willi syndrome.* (pp. 45–53). Baltimore: University Park Press.

Hasegawa, T., Hara, M., Ando, M., Osawa, M., Fukuyama, Y., Takahasi, M., & Yamada, K. (1984). Cytogenetic studies of familial Prader-Willi syndrome. *Human Genetics, 65,* 325–330.

Hawkey, C. J., & Smithies, A. (1976). The Prader-Willi syndrome with a 15/15 translocation: Case report and review of the literature. *Journal of Medical Genetics, 13,* 152–156.

Hittner, H. M., Riccardi, V. M., & Francke, U. (1979). Anirdia caused by a heritable chromosome 11 deletion. *Ophthalmology, 86,* 1176–1183.

Hobbins, J. C., Grannum, P. A., Romero, R., Reece, E. A., & Mahoney, M. J. (1985). Percutaneous umbilical blood sampling. *American Journal of Obstetrics and Gynecology 152,* 1–6.

Holm, V. A. (1981). The diagnosis of Prader-Willi syndrome. In: V. A. Holm, S. Sulzbacher, & P. L. Pipes (Eds), *Prader-Willi syndrome.* (pp. 27–44). Baltimore: University Park Press.

International Fetoscopy Group (1984). Special report: The status of fetoscopy and fetal tissue sampling. *Prenatal Diagnosis, 4,* 79–81.

Kousseff, B. G. (1982). The cytogenetic controversy in the Prader-Labhart-Willi syndrome. *American Journal of Medical Genetics, 13,* 431–439.

Kousseff, B. G., & Agatucci, A. (1981). Aniridia-Wilms tumor association. *The Journal of Pediatrics, 98,* 676–677.

Labidi, F., & Cassidy, S. B. (1986). A blind prometaphase study of Prader-Willi syndrome: Frequency and consistency in interpretation of del 15q. *American Journal of Human Genetics, 39,* 452–460.

Laurance, B. M., Brito, A., & Wilkinson, J. (1981). Prader-Willi syndrome after age 15 years. *Archives of Diseases in Childhood, 56,* 181–186.

Ledbetter, D. H., Riccardi, V. M., Airhart, S. D., Strobel, R. J., Keenan, B. S., & Crawford, J. D. (1981). Deletions of chromosome 15 as a cause of the Prader-Willi syndrome. *The New England Journal of Medicine, 304,* 325–329.

Ledbetter, D. H., Mascarello, J. T., Riccardi, V. M., Harper, V. D., Airhart, S. D., & Strobel, R. J. (1982). Chromosome 15 abnormalities and the Prader-Willi syndrome: A follow-up report of 40 cases. *American Journal of Human Genetics, 34,* 278–285.

Lejeune, J., Maunoury, C., Prieur, M., & van den Akker, J. (1979). Translocation sauteuse (5p;15q), (8q;15q), (12q;15q). *Annales de Genetique, 22,* 210–213.

Mattei, J. F., Mattei, M. G., & Giraud, F. (1983). Prader-Willi syndrome and chromosome 15: A clinical discussion of 20 cases. *Human Genetics, 64,* 356–362.

Mattei, M. G., Souiah, N., & Mattei, J. F. (1984). Chromosome 15 anomalies and the Prader-Willi syndrome: Cytogenetic analysis. *Human Genetics, 66,* 313–334.

Niebuhr, E. (1978). The cri du chat syndrome. *Human Genetics, 44,* 227–275.

Niikawa, N., & Ishikiriyama, S. (1985). Clinical and cytogenetic studies of the

Prader-Willi syndrome: Evidence of phenotype-karyotype correlation. *Human Genetics 69,* 22–27.

Prader, A., Labhart, A., & Willi, H. (1956). Ein syndrom von adipositas, kleinwuchs, kryptorchismus und oligophrenie nach myatonieartigem zustand in neugeborenalter. *Schweizerische Medizinische Wochenschrift, 86,* 1260–1261.

Rivera, H., Turleau, C., de Grouchy, J., Junien, C., Despoisse, S., & Zucker, J-M. (1981). Retinoblastoma-del (13q14): Report of two patients, one with a trisomic sib due to maternal insertion. Gene-dosage effect for esterase D. *Human Genetics, 59,* 211–214.

Schinzel, A. (1986). Approaches to the prenatal diagnosis of the Prader-Willi syndrome. *Human Genetics, 74,* 327.

Smith, A., & Noel M. (1980). A girl with the Prader-Willi syndrome and Robertsonian translocation 45,XX,t(14;15)(p11;q11) which was present in three normal family members. *Human Genetics 55,* 271–273.

Strong, L. C., Riccardi, V. M., Ferrell, R. E., & Sparkes, R. S. (1981). Familial retinoblastoma and chromosome 13 deletion transmited via an insertional translocation. *Science, 213,* 1501–1503.

Takano, T., Nakagome, Y., Nagafuchi, S., Tanaka, F., Nakamura, Y., Nagano, T., Tanae, A., & Hibi, I. (1986). High-resolution cytogenetic studies in patients with Prader-Willi syndrome. *Clinical Genetics, 30,* 241–248.

Wu, R. H., Hasen, J., & Warburton, D. (1981). Primary hypogonadism and 13/15 chromosome translocation in Prader-Labhart-Willi syndrome. *Hormone Research, 15,* 148–158.

Yunis, J. J. (1976). High resolution of human chromosomes. *Science, 191,* 1268–1270.

Yunis, J. J., & Ramsay, N. K. C. (1980). Familial occurrence of the aniridia-Wilms tumor syndrome with deletion 11p13-14.1. *The Journal of Pediatrics, 96,* 1027–1030.

Zellweger, H., & Schneider, H. J. (1968). Syndrome of hypotonia-hypomentia-hypogonadism-obesity (HHHO), or Prader-Willi syndrome. *American Journal of Diseases of Childhood, 115,* 588–598.

3
Cognitive and Behavioral Characteristics

RONALD L. TAYLOR

Even though there has been more familiarity with diagnostic methods and more available information regarding etiology, Prader-Willi syndrome has remained essentially a clinical phenotype. The majority of the characteristics of Prader-Willi syndrome that delineate it from other conditions are medically related. For example, hypotonia, short stature, and cryptorchidism are all frequently reported (see Chapter 1). There are, however, several nonmedical characteristics that are reported in the literature as being associated with the syndrome. These generally fall into the areas of cognition, adaptive/maladaptive behavior, and food-related behavior.

Cognition

Perhaps the most widely accepted definition of mental retardation is that of the American Association on Mental Deficiency (AAMD; Grossman, 1983). That definition and associated classification system was recently modified to provide more consistency among various nosological systems. For example, the AAMD definition is used with only slight word changes by the World Health Organization's International Classification of Diseases and the American Psychiatric Association's Diagnostic and Statistical Manual III (Warren & Taylor, 1984). That definition states that mental retardation includes both deficits in intellectual performance (70–75 as the upper limit) *and* deficits in adaptive behavior. Despite the AAMD's classification system, a number of different definitions are still used, and it is often unclear which definition is being used when individuals are labeled as retarded (Taylor, 1980).

When Prader-Willi syndrome was first described, hypomentia, or mental retardation, was a reported characteristic (Prader, Labhart, & Willi, 1956). Later, Zellweger and Schneider (1968) referred to Prader-Willi syndrome as the Hypotonia-Hypomentia-Hypogonadism-Obesity (HHHO) syndrome, again suggesting that mental retardation was one of the identifying features. It is important to note, however, that these and most other reports were looking more at intellectual performance than at a combination of intellectual and adaptive behavior skills, and that it was unclear which definition of mental retardation was being used.

Until recently, it has been assumed that the majority of individuals with Prader-Willi syndrome fall into the retarded range of intellectual development. For example, Hall and Smith (1972) reported that all but 1 of 32 subjects studied were mentally deficient. The average IQ of their subjects was 55, although the IQs ranged from 18 to within the normal limits. Smith (1976) noted that the IQs of individuals with the syndrome were usually between 20 and 80, with the majority falling between 40 and 60. Jancar (1971) reported IQs ranging from 12 to 42. These reports led to a general consensus that the vast majority of individuals with Prader-Willi syndrome was retarded. Some investigators (e.g., Bahling, 1979), in fact, made inappropriate generalizations about individuals with the syndrome, stating that most are profoundly retarded.

More recently, evidence has indicated that while some degree of cognitive differences is usually present, as many as 50% of the population has intelligence test scores that place them outside the retarded range (e.g., Holm, 1981). Holm noted the results of a questionnaire in which 12% of the sample of Prader-Willi individuals was reported to be in the normal range and 29% in the borderline range of intelligence. In a recent study, Taylor and Caldwell (1985) individually administered the Weschler Adult Intelligence Scale to 12 individuals with the syndrome and found that 50% had IQs outside the retarded range (average IQ = 70.25). There have been isolated reports of IQs over 100 (e.g., Crnic, Sulzbacher, Snow, & Holm, 1980). The reasons for the higher reported IQs in recent years are unclear. One possible explanation is the placement of more individuals with Prader-Willi syndrome into more appropriate educational programs. Many of these individuals have only recently been given the type of regular or special education placement that would foster cognitive growth. Another explanation is the development of improved diagnostic procedures and the subsequent greater recognition of the syndrome. In other words, as the syndrome becomes publicized and the diagnostic information more widespread, more children with Prader-Willi syndrome are being identified. In the earlier years, perhaps only the more severe cases were diagnosed. Still another explanation is that children with the syndrome are being identified earlier. As will be discussed next, there is some evidence that measured intelligence decreases with age for children with Prader-Willi syndrome.

In addition to the *levels* of cognitive ability, two other issues seem to be widespread in the discussion of intellectual development. As noted, the first relates to evidence suggesting that IQ decreases during the early years (Dunn, 1968), particularly between the ages of 6 and 10 (Dunn, Tze, Alisharan, & Schulzer, 1981). The reasons for this decline is unclear. For instance, Krywaniak (1977) noted that for those individuals with Prader-Willi syndrome who were institutionalized, the declining IQ with age is not surprising. Perhaps the most logical explanation, however, is regression in IQ relative to age norms, a statistical phenomenon that is certainly not new. For example, the decrease in IQ among individuals with Down syndrome is well documented (e.g., Macmillan, 1983; Robinson & Robinson, 1976). A distinction between *statistical* regression and *clinical* regression must, therefore, be made. That a child's IQ decreases over time does not imply that the child is losing cognitive skills as he/she gets older. In fact most of these children learn a significant amount of information and become more competent in daily living skills. Rather, this decrease in IQ suggests that as the child with a cognitive problem gets older, the discrepancy between his/her performance and "average" preformance (of the standardization sample on which IQs are based) gets larger. For one thing, as a child gets older, his/her IQ is determined based on more and varied tasks. This could explain the greater decline in IQ between the ages of 6 and 10. We also know that intelligence test scores in the "normal" population can fluctuate significantly over time (Reschly, 1979; Taylor, 1984). Among other reasons this fluctuation could be due to a variety of educational and environmental experiences. Another factor could be test selection. Some developmental measure typically is used between birth and ages 3 to 4. After this age, more traditional intelligence measures are used that include problem solving and other conceptual tasks. Therefore, instrument differences also could account for the differences in IQs as a function of age.

Another related cognitive issue was reported by Crnic et al. (1980). They concluded that IQ also declined with increased weight. In other words, the more obese the individual, the slower the rate of cognitive development. Unfortunately, such correlational data cannot be interpreted in a cause and effect framework, and the possible meaning of, as well as the reasons for, the relationship between increased obesity and lowered IQ is highly debatable. Crnic et al. (1980) noted, for instance, that when their subjects lost weight their IQs did not subsequently increase. They suggested that early factors of brain development (e.g., myelination) might be involved. They also indicated the possibility of other explanations such as limited mobility or negative psychosocial factors related to the obesity, a point that should not be overlooked. Clearly more data are needed in this area before definitive statements can be made.

Another area of controversy is centered around the *pattern* of cognitive deficits demonstrated by individuals with Prader-Willi syndrome. Although Holm (1981) stated that "there is no typical cognitive developmental pattern in Prader-Willi syndrome" (pp. 32–33), several characteristic strengths and weaknesses are associated with the syndrome. Hanson (1981) noted that there was a characteristic pattern of deficits in short-term memory and the processing of visual information. Warren and Hunt (1981) experimentally determined that individuals with Prader-Willi syndrome had poorer picture recognition memory than did undifferentiated retarded subjects. They concluded that individuals with Prader-Willi syndrome had greater short-term memory processing problems than retarded individuals without the syndrome. They also noted that their data did not support greater long-term memory problems for Prader-Willi syndrome children.

Interestingly, one area of reported strength has been visual analysis or puzzle-solving ability (Holm, 1981). Landwirth, Schwartz, and Grunt (1968), however, noted in a case report that their subject demonstrated consistent perceptual deficits even in the presence of normal-to-low average intelligence. This latter report, along with Warren and Hunt's finding of visual processing problems, suggests that the area of visual-perception/visual-motor integration cannot be regarded as a skill area that is consistently strong or weak for these individuals.

In a series of studies, the cognitive strengths and weaknesses of individuals with Prader-Willi syndrome were determined and compared with the patterns of a group of obese individuals without the syndrome who were functioning at a similar overall cognitive level (Taylor & Caldwell, 1983). They found that their studies supported the majority of the cognitive strengths and deficits reported in the literature. (See Table 3.1.) For example, three of the Prader-Willi syndrome groups' highest scores were in areas of visual perception, visual organization, and puzzle solving. They also found that verbal skills were slightly de-

TABLE 3.1. Results of the Wechsler Adult Intelligence Scale.

Scale/subtest	Prader-Willi		Non-Prader-Willi		
	$\bar{X}^a$	SD	$\bar{X}$	SD	F
Full-scale IQ	70.25	9.33	65.00	14.02	1.17
Verbal IQ	70.17	7.55	66.00	15.32	.71
Performance IQ	74.67	12.64	68.17	12.14	1.65
Information	3.92	1.16	3.92	1.98	.005
Similarities	7.67	3.06	5.83	3.61	1.80
Vocabulary	4.00	1.76	4.50	2.75	.28
Arithmetic	3.83	1.03	3.33	2.84	.33
Comprehension	4.58	1.98	4.33	3.28	.05
Digit span	3.92	2.84	2.50	3.06	1.38
Picture completion	6.83	1.11	6.17	2.12	.93
Picture arrangement	5.17	3.59	4.42	2.81	.32
Block design	7.25	2.67	4.92	1.98	5.93*
Object assembly	6.33	2.02	5.25	2.26	1.54
Digit symbol	4.83	3.16	4.33	2.46	.19

[a]Scores presented are IQs and subtest scaled scores.
*$p < .05$.

pressed compared with nonverbal skills. This is inconsistent with previous reports that note language strengths in this population (Holm, 1981). The lowest nonverbal area was a task requiring a certain degree of visual memory, a finding consistent with that of Warren and Hunt (1981). Interestingly, however, there were very few statistical differences between the Prader-Willi and non-Prader-Willi group; the patterns were, in fact, very similar. For example, the lowest area for both groups was rote short-term auditory memory. The only area in which there were statistical differences was visual organization skills in which the Prader-Willi group was superior. It appears, therefore, that *several of the reported cognitive characteristics of Prader-Willi syndrome are present, although they do not appear necessarily to be unique to the syndrome itself.*

Other investigators such as Sulzbacher, Crnic, and Snow (1981) have noted that individuals with Prader-Willi syndrome have standardized test profiles that are more consistent with learning disabled than mentally retarded individuals. They went on to state that they have significant problems with math and much less difficulty with reading. Holm (1981), in the results of a questionnaire, also noted that they were better in reading than in math. She also found that the respondents indicated that the academic performances of Prader-Willi individuals are less than expected for their IQ level. In testing these characteristics, Taylor and Caldwell (1983) found that reading scores on a standardized achievement test were slightly higher (standard score 73) than their math scores (standard score 70). Again there were no differences between the Prader-Willi and non-Prader-Willi syndrome groups in reading, spelling, or math. They also found, however, that the subjects performed at an academic level fairly consistent with their IQ level (mean IQ = 70.25). In other words, their relative scores (compared with the standardization samples) were about the same on both intelligence and achievement measures.

In summary, it seems that many of the reported characteristics of Prader-Willi syndrome might not be unique to the syndrome. Although there is some conflicting information in this area, it would seem inappropriate at this time to assume that these characteristics are associated *only* with Prader-Willi syndrome. Many of these characteristics are found in obese, handicapped populations without the syndrome. Interindividual differences among Prader-Willi individuals and the general lack of support for finding typical patterns of performances of other populations (e.g., learning disabled) reinforces this notion (e.g., Taylor, Ziegler, & Partenio, 1984; Taylor, Partenio, & Ziegler, 1985).

Adaptive and Maladaptive Behavior

Another area in which there is a number of nonmedical characteristics reported in the literature is that of adaptive and maladaptive behavior.

The majority of the maladaptive characteristics falls into the general category of severe temper tantrums and aggressive behavior. Hall and Smith (1972) reported that serious personality problems occurred in most individuals with Prader-Willi syndrome by the time they reach adolescence and adulthood. They noted that 71% of the 32 subjects they followed had some type of personality problems and acted violently with limited provocation. They also noted that the subjects were depressed frequently. Zellweger and Schneider (1968) also noted that severe tantrums and rage reactions were associated with the syndrome. Hanson (1981) noted that while temper tantrums were associated with Prader-Willi syndrome, most individuals with the syndrome were also described as friendly, cheerful, and good-natured.

In one study attempting to compare the behavioral characteristics of Prader-Willi syndrome with a control group, Turner and Ruvalcaba (1981) investigated the recorded behavior of 10 Prader-Willi and 10 non-Prader-Willi institutionalized subjects (mean IQ ~ 45). They found that the Prader-Willi subjects were more verbally aggressive, self-abusive, and regressive than the institutionalized control subjects. The control group, however, showed more inappropriate sexual behavior. Unfortunately the length of institutionalization was not controlled in this study so it is difficult to determine what if any effect this variable had on the findings. Another methodological flaw in this study was the lack of reliability of information regarding the behavioral reports. The criteria used for determining inappropriate behavior were not stated and the amount of agreement found among the raters was not clear.

Another associated characteristic is self-abusive behavior, particularly in the form of picking and scratching (Hanson, 1981). Taylor and Caldwell (1983) noted, for example, that individuals with Prader-Willi syndrome had test scores on the AAMD Adaptive Behavior Scale indicating that they engaged in significantly more self-abusive behavior than a handicapped, obese, non-Prader-Willi syndrome comparison group (see Table 3.2).

Emotional lability, or the vacillation of emotional state, also is associated with Prader-Willi syndrome. This lability has been likened to that of learning disabled individuals (Sulzbacher, Crnic, and Snow, 1981). They also noted that individuals with Prader-Willi syndrome had poor social relationships with parents, peers, and teachers, which are sometimes associated with a poor self-concept. Interestingly, they cited Johnson (1972) who noted that this problem (picking up social cues) was certainly not unique to children with Prader-Willi syndrome, but to a certain degree seemed to be a problem for all children.

In the area of adaptive behavior, individuals with Prader-Willi syndrome are thought to have strengths in the area of feeding and meal preparation, relative strengths in dressing and grooming, but weaknesses in areas such as time and number concepts (Holm, 1981). Taylor and

TABLE 3.2. Results of the American Association on Mental Deficiency Adaptive Behavior Scale.

Part/domain	Prader-Willi		Non-Prader-Willi		
	$\bar{X}^a$	SD	$\bar{X}$	SD	F
Part I					
Independent functioning	64.42	25.04	57.67	24.89	.44
Physical development	43.25	28.42	67.67	26.45	4.75*
Economic activity	78/42	19.14	72.92	14.97	.61
Language development	78.53	22.21	78.42	13.91	.0003
Numbers and time	75.58	28.53	87.92	17.83	1.61
Domestic activity	78.58	18.59	71.08	13.54	1.28
Vocational activity	63.08	32.11	69.83	26.56	.31
Self-direction	56.67	26.97	52.00	23.86	.20
Responsibility	73.17	20.41	66.00	22.43	.67
Socialization	75.08	29.17	65.08	25.17	.81
Part II					
Violent and destructive behavior	58.25	16.10	52.17	15.64	.88
Antisocial behavior	60.25	19.42	61.50	25.46	.02
Rebellious behavior	61.58	19.44	70.17	23.70	.94
Untrustworthy behavior	63.25	10.49	73.75	18.16	3.01
Withdrawal	65.33	17.22	64.08	14.88	.04
Stereotyped behavior	63.58	5.42	68.33	10.08	2.07
Inappropriate interpersonal mannerisms	72.58	8.76	72.33	6.60	.006
Unacceptable vocal habits	71.25	8.76	76.17	10.89	1.49
Unacceptable or eccentric habits	66.67	10.94	66.25	9.80	.008
Self-abusive behavior	81.42	9.89	73.92	4.40	5.76*
Hyperactive tendencies	73.33	7.40	75.17	10.28	.25
Sexually aberrant behavior	68.00	6.42	71.92	7.93	1.77
Psychological disturbances	63.08	22.15	64.00	23.42	.009
Use of medications	54.83	9.93	57.08	13.73	.21

[a]Scores presented are percentiles.
*$p < .05$.

Caldwell (1983) found that a sample of individuals with Prader-Willi syndrome scored the lowest in the areas of physical development and self-direction. Although they scored slightly lower than did the comparison group on numbers and time, there were no significant differences. In fact, the Prader-Willi and non-Prader-Willi groups scored very similarly in all areas but physical development (see Table 3.2).

FOOD-RELATED BEHAVIOR

Because obesity is such a pervasive characteristic of Prader-Willi syndrome, it is not surprising that food-related behaviors are a focus of considerable attention. Unfortunately, much of this attention has been placed on the more "sensationalist" aspects such as the eating of unacceptable products including garbage, animal food, and frozen food (e.g., Coplin, Hine, & Gormican, 1976). Two other characteristics frequently mentioned are food obsession and stealing (e.g., Holm & Pipes, 1976; Zellweger & Schneider, 1968). Two issues should be discussed regarding these aberrant food-related behaviors. The first concerns the generalization of these reports. In other words, how safe can we be in stating that these behaviors are characteristic of all individuals with the syndrome? The second involves an analysis of the environmental factors that could lead to these behaviors.

The implication one receives in reading accounts (particularly aimed toward lay people), of Prader-Willi syndrome is that the unusual food-related behaviors are the hallmark of the syndrome. Both the degree and frequency of this particular aspect of Prader-Willi syndrome, like many others, have been overgeneralized. While it is true that there have been numerous reports of unacceptable food-related behavior, it does not necessarily mean that all individuals with the syndrome will display these behaviors, nor that the individuals who do display them do so all the time. These types of reports have been overgeneralized to the point where these type of behaviors are almost expected.

One must also analyze the environmental factors that play important roles in the food-related behaviors of individuals with Prader-Willi syndrome. Many individuals (e.g., Pipes & Holm, 1973) have stated that the obesity found in the syndrome is unamenable to dietary therapy and that food must be made inaccessible to those individuals. This has resulted in a highly restricted environment in which food is typically locked in cabinets and refrigerators. It is possible that many of the reported inappropriate behaviors (e.g., stealing, gorging) could be a function of this environmental factor. When the individual with Prader-Willi syndrome (or any other individual for that matter) is deprived of appropriate access to food, *any* behavior by that individual to gain access is deemed inappropriate (i.e., stealing). Individuals with Prader-Willi syndrome might *gorge* because they never know when they will gain access to food again. They might *eat unacceptable products* when they can't gain access to acceptable food products. It does not mean that they necessarily prefer such products over more appropriate and acceptable food.

The previous discussion implies that it is possible that many of the inappropriate food-related behaviors are *learned* and therefore are not a unique aspect of this syndrome. It is possible that they are a "normal" response to an "abnormal" environment, or might be indicative of any person with a food-related disorder (e.g., bulimics who binge after denying themselves access to food). Although no empirical research that specifically addresses this issue was found, observations documented during summer programs for over 8 years have indicated that when obese individuals with and without Prader-Willi syndrome are given appropriate access to food, the frequency and degree of inappropriate food-related behavior decrease. It is certainly worthy of further investigation.

Several food-related aspects of Prader-Willi syndrome have been investigated, most notably their apparent lack of food preferences (e.g., Pipes & Holm, 1973). This assumption has led to dietary programs that have emphasized the greatest *volume* of food (within certain caloric limitations). In a series of empirical studies (Caldwell & Taylor, 1983; Taylor & Caldwell, 1985), the issue of food preference among individuals with Prader-Willi syndrome was specifically investigated. From these studies, several interesting (and somewhat surprising) findings emerged. Among them were:

1. Individuals with Prader-Willi syndrome indicated a definite and, in fact, consistent food preference. All of those who demonstrated a preference chose sweet over plain, salty, or sour foods. Interestingly, this is the same preference found in the general population.
2. The degree of food preference is positively related to level of cognitive ability; the higher the cognitive level, the greater the food preference.
3. Individuals with the syndrome consistently chose a lesser amount of their preferred food over a greater amount (twice as much) of their non-preferred food.
4. It appears that low-calorie sweets (those containing sugar substitutes) can be used in place of high-calorie foods containing sugar without affecting their preference to a marked degree.

These findings have many potential implications for dietary and weight management programs. First, they suggest that preferential food should be incorporated into the dietary program of individuals with the syndrome. Since they chose to eat a lesser amount of their preferred food over twice the amount of their nonpreferred food, it seems only reasonable to allow some choice in their menu, while still remaining at the same caloric level. *If* some of the inappropriate food-related behavior is learned, then such a change in dietary programming could have a positive effect. For example, if individuals are always deprived of certain foods, it only makes sense that they would gorge themselves when they gain access to those foods.

A second implication is that some food-related behavior of individuals with Prader-Willi syndrome may be more a function of level of cognitive ability than the syndrome per se. All of the nonretarded subjects in the study demonstrated a preference for sweet foods. The retarded subjects, however, were less clear about their food choices. Many of these individuals responded in a manner consistent with the over-all literature on mental retardation. This included stimulus-bound positional responses when asked to choose their food samples.

It is also possible that sugar-free substitutes could be used in place of high-calorie sweet foods. This way, the individual with Prader-Willi syndrome could have both preferential food *and* a greater volume within certain limitations.

Finally, the consistent finding of food preference suggests the possibility of some type of contingent weight management program. For example, it is possible that preferred food could be made contingent on increased exercise. By adjusting the caloric intake-output ratio, it would be possible to use such a system for weight loss and/or weight management. This possibility was explored recently during a 6 week residential summer program (Caldwell, Taylor, & Bloom, 1986). In this study, 11 individuals with Prader-Willi syndrome were evaluated to determine most and least preferred foods. All of the subjects chose high-calorie snacks (e.g., cookies, candy) over traditional diet foods (e.g., celery, carrot). The next part of the experiment offered each individual the opportunity to perform 20 minutes of a prescribed activity (e.g., walking, bicycling) under three experimental conditions: no reinforcement, reinforcement in the form of low-preference food, and reinforcement in the form of high-preference food. Seven of the eleven subjects increased their activity level and five of those seven only increased during the high-preference condition (see Figure 3.1).

There are at least two implications of these findings. First, contrary to many previous reports, the individuals demonstrated consistent food preferences. Secondly, the caloric expenditure for the 20 minutes of exercise was *greater* than the caloric intake for the reinforcer. Thus, in addition to the physical benefits of the exercise (e.g., increased cardiovascular efficiency), there was a net decrease in calories.

Summary

There has been a number of cognitive and behavioral characteristics traditionally associated with Prader-Willi syndrome. Many of these characteristics have been based on observation, parent reports, and early descriptions of the syndrome. As more information becomes available about Prader-Willi syndrome, many of these characteristics are challenged. In the area of cognition, for example, the earlier reports that the vast majority of individuals with the syndrome are mentally retarded has been refuted by recent empirical evidence. Other characteristics (e.g., decreased IQ with increased age and increased obesity) are subject to alternative explanations that are not related to Prader-Willi syndrome. Still other characteristics, such as short-term auditory memory deficits, while associated with Prader-Willi syndrome, are also associated with similar handicapped, obese individuals without Prader-Willi syndrome. Thus many of the characteristics are not *unique* to Prader-Willi syndrome.

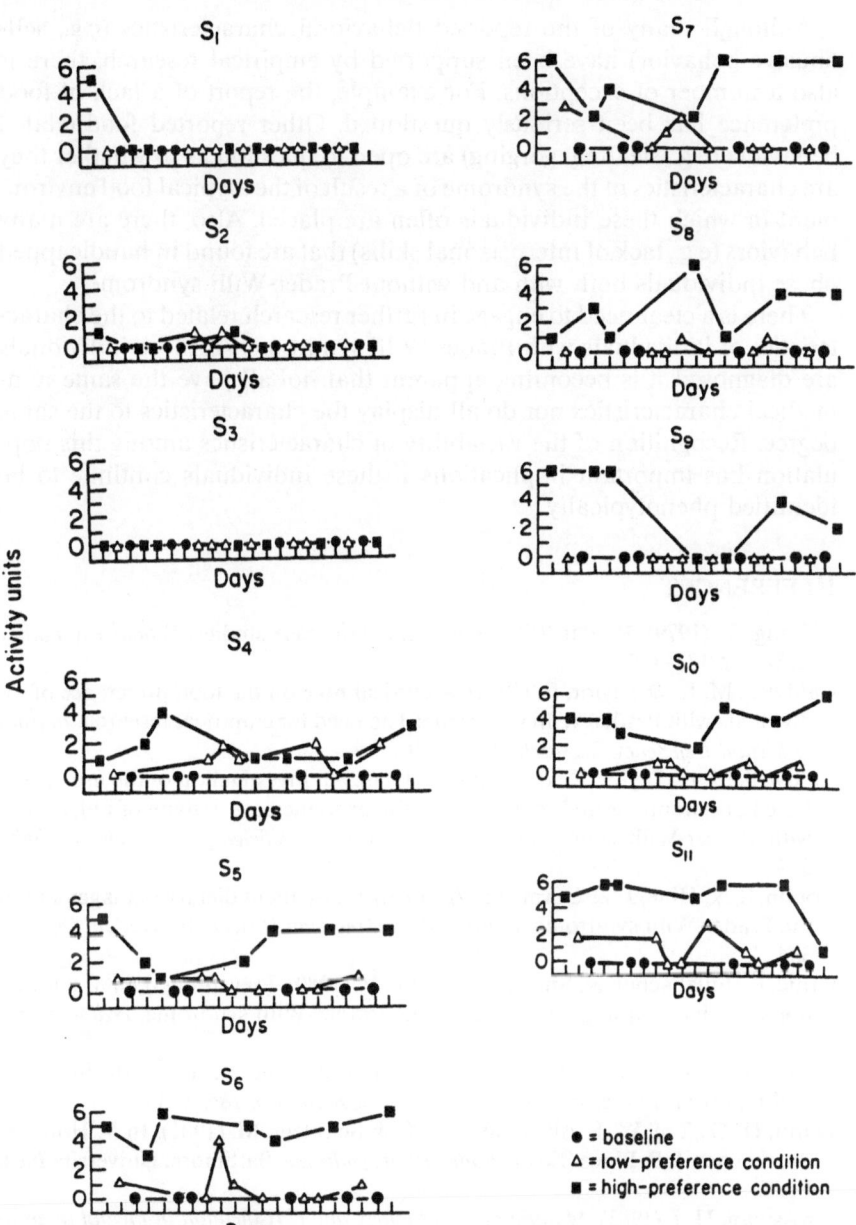

FIGURE 3.1. Activity gained for three conditions. Subjects 1, 2, and 3 showed little or no effect, no clear effects were noted for subject 4, high-preference food was effective for subjects 5, 6, 7, 8, and 9, while high-preference and, to a lesser degree, low-preference food was effective for subjects 10 and 11.

Although many of the reported behavioral characteristics (e.g., self-abusive behavior) have been supported by empirical research, there is also a number of exceptions. For example, the report of a lack of food preference has been seriously questioned. Other reported food-related behaviors (e.g., stealing, gorging) are open to question as to whether they are characteristics of the syndrome or a result of the atypical food environment in which these individuals often are placed. Also, there are many behaviors (e.g., lack of interpersonal skills) that are found in handicapped obese individuals both with and without Prader-Willi syndrome.

There is a clear need to engage in further research related to the characteristics of individuals with Prader-Willi syndrome. As more individuals are diagnosed it is becoming apparent that not all have the same non-medical characteristics nor do all display the characteristics to the same degree. Recognition of the variability of characteristics among this population has important implications if these individuals continue to be identified phenotypically.

REFERENCES

Bahling, E. (1979). Prader-Willi syndrome: Two case studies. *School Psychology Review, 8,* 133–136.

Caldwell, M. L., & Taylor, R. (1983). A clinical note on the food preference of individuals with Prader-Willi syndrome: The need for empirical research. *Journal of Mental Deficiency Research, 27,* 45–49.

Caldwell, M. L., Taylor, R., & Bloom, S. (1986). An investigation of the use of preferred and nonpreferred food as a reinforcer to increase activity of individuals with Prader-Willi syndrome. *Journal of Mental Deficiency Research, 30,* 347–354.

Coplin, S. S., Hine, J., & Gormican, A. (1976). Out-patient dietary management in the Prader-Willi syndrome. *Journal of the American Dietetic Association, 68,* 330–334.

Crnic, K., Sulzbacher, S., Snow, J., & Holm, V. (1980). Preventing mental retardation associated with gross obesity in the Prader-Willi syndrome. *Pediatrics, 66,* 787–789.

Dunn, H. G. (1968). The Prader-Labhart-Willi syndrome: Review of the literature and report of nine cases. *Acta Paediatrica Scandinavia, 186,* 1–38.

Dunn, H. G., Tze, W. J., Alisharan, R. M., & Schulzer, M. (1981). In V. Holm, S. Sulzbacher, & P. Pipes (Eds.), *Prader-Willi syndrome.* Baltimore: University Park Press.

Grossman, H. J. (1983). *Manual on terminology and classification in mental retardation.* Washington, DC: American Association on Mental Deficiency.

Hall, B. D., & Smith, D. W. (1972). Prader-Willi syndrome: A resume of 32 cases including an instance of affected first cousins, one of whom is of normal stature and intelligence. *Pediatrics, 81,* 286–293.

Hanson, J. (1981). A view of the etiology and pathogenesis of Prader-Willi syndrome. In V. Holm, S. Sulzbacher, & P. Pipes (Eds.) *Prader-Willi syndrome.* Baltimore: University Park Press.

Holm, V. (1981). The diagnosis of Prader-Willi syndrome. In V. Holm, S. Sulzbacher, & P. Pipes (Eds.) *Prader-Willi syndrome.* Baltimore: University Park Press.

Holm, V., & Pipes, P. (1976). Food and children with Prader-Willi syndrome. *American Journal of the Diseases of Children, 130,* 1063–1067.

Jancar, J. (1971). Prader-Willi syndrome (hypotonia, obesity, hypogonadism, growth and mental retardation). *Journal of Mental Deficiency Research, 15,* 20–29.

Johnson, D. (1972). *Reaching out.* Englewood Cliffs, NJ: Prentice-Hall.

Krywaniak, L. (1977). The Prader-Willi syndrome. *Mental Retardation Bulletin, 5,* 30–33.

Landwirth, J., Schwartz, A. H., & Grunt, J. A. (1968). Prader-Willi syndrome. *American Journal of Diseases of Children, 116,* 211–217.

MacMillan, D. (1983). *Mental retardation in school and society* (2nd Ed.). Boston: Little Brown.

Pipes, P., & Holm, V. (1973). Weight control of children with Prader-Willi syndrome. *Journal of the American Dietetic Association, 62,* 520–524.

Prader, A., Labhart, A., & Willi, H. (1956). Ein syndrom von Adipositas, Kleinwuchs, Kryptochismus and oligophrenie nach myatonieartigem Zustand in Neugeborenenaltar. *Schweizerische Medizinische Wochenschrift, 86,* 1260–1261.

Reschly, D. (1979). Nonbiased assessment. In G. Phye, & D. Reschly (Eds.), *School psychology: Perspectives and issues.* New York: Academic Press.

Robinson, N., & Robinson, H. (1976). *The mentally retarded child* (2nd ed.). New York: McGraw-Hill.

Smith, D. (1976). *Recognizable patterns of human malformation: Genetic, embryologic, and clinical aspects* (2nd ed.). Philadelphia: W. B. Saunders.

Sulzbacher, S., Crnic, K., & Snow, J. (1981). Behavioral and cognitive disabilities in Prader-Willi syndrome. In V. Holm, S. Sulzbacher, & P. Pipes (Eds.), *Prader-Willi syndrome.* Baltimore: University Park Press.

Taylor, R. (1980). Use of the AAMD classification system: A review of recent research. *American Journal of Mental Deficiency, 85,* 116–119.

Taylor, R. (1984). *Assessment of exceptional students: Educational and psychological procedures.* Englewood Cliffs, NJ: Prentice-Hall.

Taylor, R., & Caldwell, M. L. (1983). Psychometric performances of handicapped obese individuals with and without Prader-Willi syndrome. Paper presented at the meeting of the American Association on Medical Deficiency, Dallas, TX.

Taylor, R., & Caldwell, M. L. (1985). Type and magnitude of food preferences of individuals with Prader-Willi syndrome. *Journal of Mental Deficiency Research, 29,* 109–112.

Taylor, R., Partenio, I., & Ziegler, E. (1985). Diagnostic use of WISC-R subtest scatter: A note of caution. *Diagnostique, 11,* 9–13.

Taylor, R., Ziegler, E., & Partenio, I. (1984). Investigation of WISC-R verbal performance discrepancies as a function of ethnic status. *Psychology in the Schools, 21,* 436–441.

Turner, R., & Ruvalcaba, R. (1981). A retrospective study of the behavior of Prader-Willi syndrome vs. other institutionalized retarded persons. In V. Holm, S. Sulzbacher, and P. Pipes (Eds.), *Prader-Willi syndrome.* Baltimore: University Park Press.

Warren, J., & Hunt, E. (1981). Cognitive processing in children with Prader-Willi syndrome. In V. Holm, S. Sulzbacher, & P. Pipes (Eds.), *Prader-Willi syndrome.* Baltimore: University Park Press.

Warren, S. A., & Taylor, R. (1984). Educational characteristics of children with learning disorders. *The Pediatric Clinics of North America, 31,* 331–343.

Zellweger, H., & Schneider, H. (1968). Syndrome of hypotonia-hypomentia-hypogonadism-obesity (HHHO) or Prader-Willi syndrome. *American Journal of Diseases of Children, 115,* 588–598.

4
Management of the Problems of Infancy: Hypotonia, Developmental Delay, and Feeding Problems

SUZANNE B. CASSIDY

Among the various medical problems related to infants with Prader-Willi syndrome, those that have implications for management include hypotonia, developmental delay, and feeding problems.

Hypotonia and Developmental Delay

Generalized hypotonia in infancy is a consistent characteristic of Prader-Willi syndrome and one that has serious consequences. The hypotonia is present at the time of birth, resulting in "floppy infant syndrome," and is severe in the majority of cases (Zellweger, 1981). Zellweger noted, in fact, that infants and newborns with Prader-Willi syndrome present a clinical picture very similar to that seen in individuals with disorders of the lower motor unit or spinal cord, and in individuals with severe cerebral disorders. Most infants with Prader-Willi syndrome have an expressionless face, flaccid muscles, a weak cry, and little spontaneous movement. Weakness may or may not be a feature, and a good response to stimuli may be present. The infant may primarily assume the frog-leg position, with arms and legs resting on the bed flexed and abducted. Deep tendon reflexes and the Moro response are often diminished or absent (Zellweger, 1981).

The hypotonia seen in Prader-Willi syndrome is supraspinal, or central, in origin as indicated by normal neuromotor unit studies; with rare exception (Hooft, Delire, & Cosneuf, 1966) serum creatinine phosphokinase (CPK), nerve conduction velocity (NCV), and electromyography (EMG) are normal (Zellweger & Schneider, 1968). Muscle biopsy specimens have been reported to be normal in most cases (Dubowitz, 1978), although in some individuals type II fiber atrophy consistent with disuse has been seen (Zellweger, 1981). Electron microscopic studies of muscle biopsy specimens have shown the kinds of nonspecific changes also seen in essential (idiopathic) hypotonia, disuse, and neurogenic atrophy. These include aggregates of mitochondria, disruption of myofilaments, accumulation of interfibrillary debris, and irregularity of Z lines (Zellweger and Schneider, 1968; Affifi & Zellweger, 1969).

The supraspinal nature of the hypotonia is further demonstrated by the natural history of this feature in children with the syndrome. Regardless of its initial severity, the hypotonia improves and, ultimately, many of its consequences resolve. In most cases, the hypotonia is present only for the first weeks or months of life (Zellweger, 1981). Although muscle tone approaches normal, poor coordination and motor delays persist and it is rare for the person with Prader-Willi syndrome to reach normal muscular capability. As with the severity of the hypotonia, there is considerable variability as to the age and rate at which the improvement in hypotonia occurs.

The hypotonia in Prader-Willi syndrome may result in any of several frequently seen abnormalities. Prenatally, fetal movements are often more feeble and less frequent than normal. Mild polyhydramnios may result from decreased swallowing. Breech and other abnormal fetal positions are common, as are a cesarean section and nonterm delivery (Holm, 1981). As found in individuals with severe hypotonia of any cause (Smith, 1982), joint contractures may develop as a consequence of inadequate fetal movement, although this is not a common observation in Prader-Willi syndrome.

Postnatally, the most serious and consistent problem related to the hypotonia is severe feeding problems resulting from weakness of suck and a poor or absent sucking reflex. Special feeding techniques are usually required in order to provide adequate nutrition (see below), and resultant prolonged hospital stay generally is necessary. Poor weight gain ("failure to thrive") is commonly the result of the feeding difficulties. Weight is below the mean in the majority and below the third percentile in many until after age 6 months, while length is generally in the normal range during this time (Nugent and Holm, 1981).

The paucity of spontaneous movement in infants with Prader-Willi syndrome, and their described placid nature, may result in decreased interaction with care-givers. This may have physical as well as emotional and psychological consequences. Hypothermia has been described (Zellweger, 1981), although the frequency with which it is found has not been documented. Presumably, it may be related in part to lack of muscle activity and its resultant heat production, and partly to hypothalamic dysfunction. Temperature should be closely monitored in the newborn period, and hypothermia treated with warmer clothing or use of an isolette. Congenital hip dislocation is noted in a minority of patients. Its treatment is no different from that in other children, and should include referral to an orthopedist. Any infant whose head is kept in the same position with great frequency may develop plagiocephaly, or head asymmetry (Clarren, 1981), which may occur with hypotonia. If tone improves by 6 to 8 months of age, the head will be exposed to more symmetric pressures during the remaining few months of rapid head growth and will probably spontaneously improve in shape. If not, a significant cosmetic problem may result. When spontaneous improvement in head shape does not occur, treatment using a specially molded helmet may be of benefit if started by age 9 months (Clarren, 1981). In addition to plagiocephaly, lack of movement may result in development of joint contractures postnatally as well as prenatally.

Delayed motor milestones are seen in virtually all infants with Prader-Willi syndrome. While this is probably related in part to their generalized central nervous system dysfunction, hypotonia is also likely to be a strongly contributory causative factor, since infants who are hypotonic for other reasons are also delayed motorically. Several patient series indicate that the average age at which early motor milestones are achieved in Prader-Willi syndrome are as follows: independent sitting, 12 to 13 months; walking, 24 to 30 months; tricycle riding, 4.2 years (Dunn, Tze, Alisharan, & Schulzer, 1981; Hall & Smith, 1972; Holm, 1981; Prader, Labhart, & Willi, 1956).

Newborns with Prader-Willi syndrome usually lie motionless in the crib, responding little to the attentions of parents or caretakers. Often, they must be awakened at feeding times, and they may be difficult to arouse. These features, combined with the efforts necessary to provide them with adequate caloric intake, might result in psychological and emotional difficulties for the parents, although descriptions of these parent-child problems in Prader-Willi syndrome and the approach to their treatment have not been reported in the published literature. (See Chapter 7 of this volume for more information regarding parent concerns.)

The known or presumed consequences of infantile hypotonia in Prader-Willi syndrome are summarized in Table 4.1

Management of Hypotonia and Developmental Delay

Physical therapy is strongly recommended for the hypotonic infant with Prader-Willi syndrome to prevent disuse atrophy and development of contractures during the period of inactivity. Ideally, this should be instituted as soon as possible, and preferably while the infant is still in the hospital. In most nurseries the nurses can perform the therapy, generally under the guidance of a consultant physical therapist. Involvement and education of the parents concerning the importance of movement to normal growth and development will help in assuring continuation of physical therapy following discharge.

Once the child is at home, referral to a physical or occupational therapist in the community can be made. In many areas, state-supported regional early intervention programs are available, and children with Prader-Willi syndrome should be eligible since they are at risk for

TABLE 4.1. Consequences of hypotonia in Prader-Willi syndrome.

Stage of development	Characteristic
Prenatal	Diminished fetal movements
	Abnormal birth position
	Need for cesarean section
	Nonterm delivery
	Congenital contractures
Neonatal	Weak cry
	Weak suck
	Abnormal neurologic examination
	Hypothermia
	Feeding problems
	Decreased motor activity
	Plagiocephaly
	Joint contractures
	Parent-child interaction problems
Infancy and childhood	Failure to thrive
	Delayed motor development
	Poor coordination

developmental delays in all areas. If not, private physical therapists affiliated with Easter Seals organizations or hospitals also may have been trained in working with hypotonic infants. Optimally, the therapist will educate the parents and other care-givers as to the importance of and techniques for range-of-motion exercises and developmental stimulation. Specific guidelines for therapy with these infants have been outlined by Carman (1981).

Infants born with congenital contractures due to lack of movement *in utero* require more vigorous and directed physical therapy, and frequently orthopedic intervention, to treat their contractures. Frequent position changes will help avoid or treat plagiocephaly.

In addition to physical therapy, specific attention to the attainment of developmental milestones is beneficial. Enrollment in a program for infant stimulation (early intervention) is desirable. Again, these are available in many places through state-supported regional programs, usually at no cost to the family. In some areas, school systems are mandated to begin education during infancy for those with or at risk for developmental delay. If no such program is offered, a physical therapist with training in early development may be available in private or institutional practice. Local agencies for individuals with mental retardation may be of benefit in finding such therapists. Ideally, the teacher or therapist works with the parents to encourage the child along normal developmental lines while improving muscle strength, in an effort to help the child develop to the fullest potential. This also helps parents to understand their child and his or her capabilities, and allows them the opportunity to intervene in improving their child's outcome.

When trained therapists and teachers are not available, or if the degree of hypotonia and motor delay does not warrant their involvement, it is possible for the parents to work with the child without consultation in order to avoid some of the physical consequences of hypotonia. For example, movement has been shown to increase the rate of motor development (Clark, Kreutzberg, & Chee, 1977; Kantner, Clark, Allen, & Chase, 1976). A number of specific recommendations has been outlined for ways in which families can work with hypotonic infants with Prader-Willi syndrome, including slowly rolling the child, carefully bouncing the child on a knee, slow rocking, and swinging the child while holding the trunk firmly under the arms (Carman, 1981).

Management of Feeding Problems

The medical and nutritional literature is strikingly devoid of publications related to the management of feeding problems of infants with hypotonia as a result of Prader-Willi syndrome. There are, however, several logical suggestions for managing these problems. First, energetic intervention is required to avoid inadequate caloric intake by most infants with the syndrome. An infant with Prader-Willi syndrome who is able to breast-feed is unusual. Few have a sufficiently strong suck to consume adequate calories for growth without the use of special feeding techniques. Enlargement of a normal or premature nipple hole, combined with considerable time and patience on the part of the feeder, will usually permit adequate intake. It is often necessary to encourage the infant to suck by stroking the cheek or gently squeezing the cheeks together, and by assuring alertness through talking and other stimulating activities. Feeding times are long and frustrating and often are viewed as a trial by parents who attempt to feed solely by nipple. Health-care providers should give considerable encouragement to parents and other care-givers to continue in their efforts as long as the child gains weight on this regimen. The possibility of giving many small feedings rather than a few large ones may allow a more enjoyable feeding experience for both parent and child, but should be discontinued as soon as possible to avoid establishment of poor eating behavior (this point is discussed later in this chapter). In the past, some parents have fed newborns with a dropper or spoon to assure adequate caloric intake, and many have chosen to introduce cup feeding early to circumvent the inadequate suck. Any of these described methods may be used, provided that the child receives sufficient calories for growth.

In most cases, children with Prader-Willi syndrome must either complete each feeding or receive the entire feeding by gavage (Hall & Smith, 1972). Since it is commonly necessary to use gavage technique for many days or weeks, and occasionally for months, it is important for parents to learn the techniques early and participate in the infant's feeding from the beginning. It is not uncommon for babies with Prader-Willi syndrome to be discharged from the nursery while still requiring gavage to complete a feeding. Since the problems related to hypotonia and consequent poor suck are transient, gavage feeding, a relatively benign intervention, is usually successful. Gastrostomy feedings and central hyperalimentation generally have not been necessary. These procedures should be avoided if possible since they emphasize the baby's differences from normal, are invasive, or have serious potential side effects.

Whatever techniques are used to feed the infant with Prader-Willi syndrome, parental support should be an integral part of the overall management program. Parents should optimally be taught the gavage technique early, since parent participation allows nurturing instincts to have a focus. Education of the parents concerning the amount of formula that is adequate for growth will further their understanding of attention to feeding. Frequent visits to health-care providers for monitoring are beneficial and often necessary, and provide the opportunity for support, encouragement, and reinforcement of the counseling. It is often helpful to involve a psychologist, social worker, or other professional trained in understanding parenting problems, particularly when physician time is too limited or when the physician is uncomfortable with discussing these issues. With proper intervention, the parents can provide a calorically adequate diet and at the same time develop a strong and positive parent-child relationship despite the feeding problems of individuals with Prader-Will syndrome.

It is important to remember that the feeding problems of early infancy will eventually resolve and the young child will become hyperphagic. As the hypotonia and feeding problems begin to improve, the emphasis previously placed on the importance of adequate feeding should be shifted to that of prevention of obesity. Then, feedings should be given at regular times and in the same place in the home. In general, overemphasis on food should be avoided. A nutritionist should be involved early with the family and should meet with them frequently for education and explanation of the importance of averting development of poor eating habits. A behavior modification program designed to address these issues has been described by Zellweger (1981). More detailed descriptions of behavioral programs can be found in Chapter 5 of this volume.

Other Management Issues of Early Infancy

It is not often that the diagnosis of Prader-Willi syndrome is made in early infancy. When it is, the opportunities for genetic counseling to aid the parents in understanding and adapting to the diagnosis are great. The anguish of not knowing the cause of the problems seen in Prader-Willi syndrome, and the guilt which most parents assign themselves for causing these problems (Leconte, 1981), can be assuaged by appropriate genetic counseling when the diagnosis is known. The role of the genetic counselor is several-fold. First, by describing the characteristics of the disorder and its natural history, it is possible to both educate the parents and diminish their fears of the unknown. Next, by explaining what is known of the etiology of the disorder, particularly if a chromosomal deletion is present, the parents can begin to understand that they did not cause the disorder. Concerns about exposures or activities before or during the pregnancy are frequently expressed by parents who do not know the cause of their child's disabilities, and they can be reassured that these are not causally related. The lack of substantially increased recurrence risk for Prader-Willi syndrome can then be communicated, and will eventually be of some solace to them. An integral part of genetic counseling involves addressing the issues of grief, sadness, and anger that are normal feelings in parents who learn that their child is disabled. The counselor can help the parents to identify these feelings and recognize them as being normal, can help open channels of communication between the parents and other family members and friends, and can help them avoid the added guilt that parents often carry because they have these feelings. Finally, the genetic counselor can help the parents see the ways in which they and others can improve the child's condition through constructive interactions and educational input. Many physicians believe that genetic counselors only discuss recurrence risks, and this mistaken understanding can rob parents of potentially valuable information and support.

Most families find it helpful to speak with other families with a child who has Prader-Willi syndrome, both in terms of learning how to handle problems that may arise and in terms of diminishing the sense of isolation that parents of children with relatively rare disorders often feel.

Summary

Hypotonia is a consistent but transient feature of infants with Prader-Willi syndrome. There are several serious consequences of this hypotonia that cause or contribute to significant problems of infancy for children with this syndrome. These problems include abnormalities of birth position and timing, delayed motor development, and severe feeding problems with subsequent failure to thrive for a period of weeks to months.

Treatment for these problems is largely supportive in nature. Physical and occupational therapy and early educational intervention for hypotonia and developmental delay help to optimize development and muscle tone. Most vital is the management of feeding problems, which usually requires special techniques such as the use of gavage feeding or special nipples with a large hole. Considerable time and patience on the part of caregivers are usually necessary when techniques other than gavage are used. Nutritional counseling should be an integral part of the overall management of the feeding problems, as well as attention to the emotional needs of the family.

Finally, family counseling, including genetic counseling concerning Prader-Willi syndrome, can help the parents understand the disorder and adapt to its unique problems. This counseling is best instituted at the time of initial diagnosis.

REFERENCES

Affifi, A. R., & Zellweger, H. (1969). Pathology of muscular hypotonia in the Prader-Willi syndrome: Light and electron microscopic study. *Journal of the Neurological Sciences, 9,* 49–61.

Carman, P. M. (1981). Physical exercise for children and adults with Prader-Willi syndrome. In V. Holm, S. Sulzbacher, & P. Pipes (Eds.), *Prader-Willi syndrome.* Baltimore: University Park Press.

Clark, D. L., Kreutzberg, J. R., & Chee, F. K. W. (1977). Vestibular stimulation influence on motor development in infants. *Science, 196,* 1228–1229.

Clarren, S. K. (1981). Plagiocephaly and torticolis: Etiology, natural history, and helmet treatment. *Journal of Pediatrics, 98,* 92–95.

Dubowitz, V. (1978). *Muscle disorders in childhood.* London: W. B. Saunders.

Dunn, H. G., Tze, W. J., Alisharan, R. M., & Schulzer, M. (1981). Clinical experience with 23 cases of Prader-Willi syndrome. In V. Holm, S. Sulzbacher, & P. Pipes (Eds.), *Prader-Willi syndrome.* Baltimore: University Park Press.

Hall, B. D., & Smith, D. W. (1972). Prader-Willi syndrome: A resumé of 32 cases including an instance of affected first cousins, one of whom is of normal stature and intelligence. *Journal of Pediatrics, 81,* 286–293.

Holm, V. A. (1981). The diagnosis of Prader-Willi syndrome. In V. Holm, S. Sulzbacher, & P. Pipes (Eds.), *Prader-Willi syndrome.* Baltimore: University Park Press.

Hooft, C., Delire, C., & Casneuf, J. (1966). Le syndrome de Prader-Willi-Fanconi: Etude clinique, endocrinologique et cytogenetique. *Acta Paediatrica Belgica, 20,* 27–50.

Kantner, R. M., Clark, D. L., Allen, L. C., & Chase, M. F. (1976). Effects of vestibular stimulation on nystagmus response and motor performance in the developmentally delayed infant. *Physical Therapy, 56,* 414–421.

Leconte, J. M. (1981). Social work intervention strategies for families with children with Prader-Willi syndrome. In V. Holm, S. Sulzbacher, & P. Pipes (Eds.), *Prader-Willi syndrome.* Baltimore: University Park Press.

Nugent, J. K., & Holm, V. A. (1981). Physical growth in Prader-Willi syndrome. In V. Holm, S. Sulzbacher, & P. Pipes (Eds.), *Prader-Willi syndrome.* Baltimore: University Park Press.

Prader, A., Labhart, A., & Willi, H. (1956). Ein Syndrom von Adipositas, Kleinwuchs, Kryptorchismus und Oligophrenie nach Myotonicartigem Zustand in Neugeborenalter. *Schweizerische Medizinische Wochenschrift, 86,* 1260–1261.

Smith, D. W. (1982). *Recognizable patterns of human malformation* (3rd ed.). Philadelphia: W. B. Saunders.

Zellweger, H., & Schneider, H. J. (1968). Syndrome of hypomentia-hypogonadism-obesity (HHO) or Prader-Willi syndrome. *American Journal of Diseases of Children, 115,* 588–598.

Zellweger, H. (1981). Diagnosis and therapy in the first phase of Prader-Willi syndrome. In V. Holm, S. Sulzbacher, & P. Pipes (Eds.), *Prader-Willi syndrome.* Baltimore: University Park Press.

5
Behavior Management and Intervention

JAMES K. LUISELLI

Behavioral psychology has made numerous contributions to education, mental health, and related disciplines.[1] For example, behavior therapy and behavioral intervention techniques have been applied with considerable success in such areas as mental retardation (Wetherby & Baumeister, 1981), psychiatry (Hersen & Bellack, 1978), and rehabilitation (Lutzker, Martin, & Rice, 1981). A more recent development related to the area of behavior therapy is the field of behavioral medicine in which learning-based interventions are used for the treatment and management of somatic disorders (Luiselli, 1987; Varni, 1983).

Behavior modification procedures have particular relevance in the design of a comprehensive treatment plan for persons with Prader-Willi syndrome. A behaviorally oriented treatment approach can be thought of as having three components (Masek, Epstein, & Russo, 1981). First, efforts at *tertiary prevention* focus on the modification of existing dysfunctional conditions directly associated with the syndrome. The most obvious example related to Prader-Willi syndrome would be procedures to reduce body weight and percentage of fat. The next area, *secondary prevention,* is aimed at reducing/eliminating behaviors that place an individual at risk for subsequent difficulties. For instance, it has been reported that many children with Prader-Willi syndrome engage in the ingestion of nonnutritive substances or unacceptable food products. Management of this behavior becomes an important therapeutic concern since it can produce intestinal blockage, parasite infestation, and weight gain (Kanner, 1957). The third treatment component is *primary prevention,* which has as its goal the strengthening of skills and competencies to avoid the development of unhealthy conditions. For example, programs might be formulated to teach individuals with Prader-Willi syndrome to make more nutritious

---

[1]As indicated by Kazdin (1982a), the terms *behavior therapy* and *behavior modification* are, at times, differentiated on the basis of conceptual foundations, treatment techniques, and settings of implementation. Typically, however, the terms are used interchangeably as they will be in the text of this chapter.

food choices or to maintain a regular schedule of physical exercise. Finally, the wide array of behavior modification treatment techniques may be employed to control management problems frequently encountered in Prader-Willi syndrome such as food stealing, aggression, and tantruming.

The purpose of this chapter is to examine how behavior analysis and therapy procedures can be and have been utilized in the treatment of persons with Prader-Willi syndrome. Given the scope of the chapter, this information is presented as a brief overview and not as an in depth presentation of theory and outcome. The material is organized into four sections. First, basic principles and techniques of behavior analysis and therapy are reviewed. Second, studies from the behavior research literature with non-Prader-Willi individuals that focus on characteristic behaviors associated with the syndrome will be discussed. Third, the literature concerned with behavioral management of individuals with Prader-Willi syndrome will be addressed. The chapter concludes with a discussion of critical issues involved in the clinical application of behavior therapy methods.

Methodology in Behavior Analysis and Therapy

The field of behavior analysis and therapy represents one area of clinical assessment and treatment subsumed under the general category of behavioral psychology. Broadly defined, this approach consists of the application of learning principles, primarily those of operant conditioning (Skinner, 1953), to the treatment of persons with behavioral, interpersonal, and adjustment problems. Behavior analysis and therapy interventions are usually implemented in applied settings such as schools, homes, and residential facilities.

The emphasis of operant learning theory is the manipulation of antecedents and consequences in the individual's environment to affect behavior change. Consequences exert control over responding through either the *presentation* or *removal* of stimuli that are either *pleasurable* or *aversive* to the individual. The presentation of a pleasurable stimulus contingent upon a response is known as *positive reinforcement* and is intended to increase the future occurrence of that response. Efforts to increase responding are also programmed through *negative reinforcement.* A negative reinforcement procedure would consist of the removal or termination of an aversive event following the display of a specified behavior. Presentation of an aversive stimulus is defined as *punishment,* a procedure that decreases the probability of the preceding response occurring again. In addition, *time-out* may be used to decrease behavior. This procedure entails the response-contingent removal of all pleasurable stimuli for a short period of time.

Extinction is another operantly based behavior change procedure. With this approach, a consequence that is known to reinforce a particular undesired behavior is withheld systematically. Rather than purposefully presenting or removing consequent stimuli when a behavior occurs, an extinction procedure would simply require a discontinuation of existing contingent reinforcement.

Antecedents are stimuli and events that precede the occurrence of a response. These include dimensions of the physicaľ environment, social behaviors, language, etc. Through their pairing with consequent events, antecedents acquire conditioned properties so that they come to control behavior by evoking or setting the occasion for responding. It is possible to decrease behavior using antecedent events. For example, if an individual has had repeated aversive experiences (e.g., getting yelled at) in the presence of specific stimuli (e.g., a particular classroom) he will become physiologically aroused, have negative thoughts, and engage in escape responses when faced with that classroom. At the same time, antecedent stimuli can be used therapeutically to initiate desired responding. These include verbal instructions, appropriate modeling of behavior, physical prompts, or visual cues.

The concentration on antecedents and consequences characterizes the *functional analytic* approach of behavioral methodology. The purpose of a functional analysis is to determine the environmental contingencies that are reinforcing and maintaining a particular behavior. In so doing, emphasis is placed on those variables currently operating within the environment rather than on historical or internal determinants of behavior. For example, various types of maladaptive behavior are reinforced by *social consequences* in the forms of adult and peer attention. Problem behaviors also may occur because they serve to *terminate or avoid unpleasant situations.* Such a condition is observed frequently in special education students who learn to avoid high-demand instructional activities by engaging in tantrumous and acting-out responses (Carr, Newsom, & Binkoff, 1980). *Sensory consequences* represent a third variable that can reinforce maladaptive behaviors and are most commonly implicated in the display of self-stimulation and some forms of self-injury (i.e., picking the skin). Finally, *organic influences* may contribute to the emergence and exacerbation of disordered behavior. The performance of a thorough functional analysis is an essential prerequisite to treatment programming since it will determine the selection of appropriate methods of intervention.

Another defining characteristic of behavior analysis and therapy is the heavy reliance on empirical assessment and evaluation. Problems targeted for intervention are defined operationally to permit objective response measurement. The emphasis is placed on the quantification of overt, publically verifiable behaviors. It is worth noting, however, that both covert and psychophysiological responses also fall within the domain of behavioral assessment (Hersen & Bellack, 1981). In terms of evaluation, response measurement is introduced before treatment implementation in order to establish a baseline by which to determine the effects of intervention. Measurement continues throughout the process of therapeutic programming and, ideally, should continue after a program has been terminated to ensure maintenance of the behavior at acceptable levels.

Whenever possible, evaluation strategies are directed at scientifically verifying the therapeutic effects of a treatment program. Procedurally, this entails utilization of single-case research methodology (Hersen & Barlow, 1984; Kazdin, 1982b). The primary focus of this approach is the repeated measurement of the behaviors under baseline (pretreatment) and treatment conditions. Changes in measured behaviors under these conditions permit conclusions to be inferred concerning the influence of treatment (independent) variables. A variety of single-case research strategies are available including *reversal* (systematically introducing and removing treatment), *multiple baseline* (sequentially applying treatment to two or more behaviors, persons, or settings), *simultaneous treatment* (rapidly alternating two or more treatments under different stimulus conditions), and *changing criterion* (gradually altering an imposed treatment standard) designs. For a complete discussion of these procedures see Hersen and Barlow (1984).

Behavioral psychologists have been prolific in formulating and experimentally validating numerous therapeutic techniques. Table 5.1 lists commonly employed behavioral treatment procedures and a brief description of each. For purposes of explication, these procedures have been subsumed under two broad categories. These are methods used for *increasing* behaviors and methods used for *decreasing* behaviors.

TABLE 5.1. Behavioral treatment procedures.

Methods to increase behaviors	
Positive reinforcement	Contingent presentation of pleasurable consequences.
Negative reinforcement	Contingent removal of unpleasant stimuli/events.
Token economy	Rewarding desirable behaviors with secondary reinforcers (e.g., poker chips, stars) that can be exchanged for a primary reinforcer (e.g., food).
Contingency contracting	Negotiating reinforcement for desirable behaviors between two persons.
Methods to decrease behavior	
DRO	Reinforcing the absence of behavior during predetermined time periods.
DRI	Reinforcing responses that are physically incompatible with the problem behavior.
Punishment	Contingent presentation of unpleasant (aversive) consequences.
Extinction	Withholding reinforcing stimuli/events.

DRO = Differential reinforcement of other behavior; DRI = differential reinforcement of incompatible behavior.

It should be emphasized that these procedures do not constitute a simple "catalogue" of methods that are selected randomly by the clinician. Rather, as indicated previously, the choice of treatment methodology depends upon carefully determining the variables that are *presently* maintaining unwanted target behaviors or interfering with the display of desired responses. Unwanted behaviors that are occurring because they are followed by pleasurable consequences, for instance, could be modified by rearranging environmental contingencies so that these consequences are made to follow desirable rather than undesirable responses. If, however, a child's unwanted behavior was reinforced by task avoidance, treatment could focus on maintaining the child in contact with the environment, perhaps through increased reinforcement for compliance. Application of a procedure such as time-out in this case would not be indicated since it would only serve to reinforce the problem behavior.

Several additional points should be highlighted regarding behavior analysis and therapy. The first is that any program of behavioral intervention must be implemented within an environment that is geared towards the contingent reinforcement of *adaptive responding*. Clearly, the most desirable way to manage interpersonal difficulties is to teach the individual effective means of controlling his/her own behavior within the natural environment. This training should initially utilize the most benign treatment techniques. If these techniques are demonstrated to be ineffective then more invasive methods of behavioral control are instituted. This least restrictive treatment model is widely accepted by practitioners (Morris & Brown, 1983). Another important consideration is that practitioners must be concerned with the impact of treatment beyond initial, short-term effects. Such issues include generalization, therapeutic maintenance, and social acceptability (these concerns will be discussed in a later section). Finally, most clinical programs within applied behavior analysis are multicomponent rather than a single-component program. The design of so-called "treatment packages" enables the clinician to tailor the most effective management strategies to the individuality of the client, the complexity of the presenting problem(s), the environments in which the treatment will take place, and the behavior to be promoted.

Behavioral Treatment of Problems Common to Prader-Willi Syndrome

The purpose of this section is to review behavioral interventions that have been effective in treating problems common to Prader-Willi syndrome. A wide range of studies will be sampled, including adult and child populations, in order to provide a flavor of the diversity of treatment application. The studies noted in this section did not use individuals with Prader-Willi syndrome as subjects. Except where noted, however, the information and techniques should be applicable to those individuals. In a subsequent section, information specifically related to individuals with Prader-Willi syndrome will be presented.

WEIGHT REDUCTION AND REGULATION

Behavioral treatment methods have been applied extensively in the areas of weight reduction and regulation. The majority of such research has been concerned with obesity in intellectually normal adults and children. Fewer applications have been reported with developmentally handicapped populations, although programmatic efforts with this group have been increasing in recent years.

Stunkard (1982) reviewed five procedural components that constitute the "typical" behavioral treatment program for adult obesity: (1) self-monitoring, (2) establishing stimulus control over eating, (3) managing specific consummatory responses, (4) reinforcing adherence to treatment contingencies, and (5) cognitive restructuring. In the process of *self-monitoring,* individuals are required to record the types and quantities of foods consumed as well as information such as the time of day when eating occurred, the stimuli linked with consumption (e.g., location, other persons present), and associated emotional responses. The goal of establishing *stimulus control* over eating is to change antecedent features of the environment that are correlated with increased or undesired consumption. Typical manipulations in this regard include eating in a uniform location, using distinctive table settings, and stocking the home with low-calorie foods. Efforts at managing specific *consummatory responses* consist of self-control procedures such as placing utensils down between bites and counting each mouthful ingested. Frequently, these procedures are augmented by increasing an individual's awareness of the singular act of eating through attention-focusing towards the flavor of the food items, the motion of chewing, and so on. *Reinforcement for adherence* to a prescribed treatment program represents a crucial ingredient in program design. For example, a token economy may be developed such that proper implementation of each component in a program is reinforced with individual points, the accumulation of which are exchanged for access to preferred activities. Finally, *cognitive restructuring techniques* are employed to change negative self-statements (e.g., "I'm fat, I'll never lose weight," or "I have Prader-Willi syndrome and I'll always be fat") to more functional, realistic evaluations (e.g., "Losing weight is difficult but I can do it if I try hard!"). The inclusion of cognitive control strategies is a somewhat recent development in the design of behavioral weight reduction programs and reflects the growing alliance between learning theorists and cognitively oriented therapists (Mahoney, 1974).

Given the widespread use of behavior therapy in the area of adult obesity, what can be said regarding therapeutic effectiveness? In a review of the behavioral literature, Brownell (1982) summarized the outcome research on this topic and concluded that in terms of short-range results, behavioral programs have been consistently successful in producing weight loss in the magnitude of 1 to 2 pounds per week over a 10- to 12-week course of treatment. When evaluated on a long-term basis, the average weight loss after 1 year of follow-up is about 10 pounds, an outcome that compares favorably with other treatment approaches. However, as underscored by Brownell (1982), many behavior therapy programs do not include deliberate, maintenance facilitating efforts and, as a result, relatively few individuals (about 25%) continue to lose weight after treatment. As with many behavior change interventions, different procedures may be responsible for initial therapeutic effects and the maintenance of those therapy gains.

Behavioral research in childhood obesity has emerged along several tracks. Analogue and naturalistic studies have identified an obese "eating style" (Drabman, Cordua, Hammer, Jarvie, & Horton, 1979; Drabman, Hammer, & Jarvie, 1977; Keane, Geller, & Scheirer, 1981). These data demonstrate that in contrast to nonobese peers, obese children take significantly more bites of food, chew less per bite, and consume their meals more rapidly. Some therapy programs, therefore, have examined methods to decrease eating rates, establish more prolonged chewing, and reduce bite size. In one investigation, Epstein, Parker, McCoy, and McGee (1976) found that simple mealtime instructions (placing utensils on the table after each bite) coupled with praise for compliance were successful in decreasing bite rate and the quantity of food consumption in obese 7-year-old children. Another study by Epstein, Masek, and Marshall (1978) produced reductions in caloric intake among six, 5- to 6-year-old obese children using a treatment program that combined instructions, cueing, and reinforcement procedures. The program was based on a "traffic light" diet in which "red" foods were to be avoided (high caloric/low nutritional value), "yellow" foods were to be eaten with caution (high caloric/moderate nutritional value), and "green" goods were to be eaten freely (low caloric/high nutritional value). The children were instructed to eat predetermined amounts of each food category prior to meals and were reinforced with stars (exchanged for inexpensive toys) if they ate within these guidelines. In addition to the lowering of food consumption, the program was associated with reductions in weight for five of the six children.

A recent trend in behavioral weight reduction programs with children is to combine a variety of treatment techniques in a broad-based approach. To illustrate, Coates and Thoresen (1981) included the following procedures in a treatment regimen with two, obese adolescent girls: (1) self-observation, (2) environmental stimulus control, (3) nutrition education, (4) self-instruction training, (5) contracting for self-selected rewards, (6) cognitive restructuring, (7) familial social support, (8) exercise participation, and (9) problem solving. As a result of intervention, weight losses of 11.5 and 21 pounds were achieved. Another component associated with significant weight reduction in obese children is having parents participate in treatment (Epstein, Wing, Koeske, Ossip, & Beck, 1982). The development of these multifaceted, "ecobehavioral" programs reflects the contemporary view among behavior weight reduction specialists that problems in weight regulation stem from multiple influences (learning, physiological, cognitive, socioenvironmental) rather than a singular etiology (Brownell, 1982; Stunkard, 1982).

Of particular relevance to the treatment of many individuals with Prader-Willi syndrome is the design of weight modification programs with developmentally disabled persons. Programs established by Fox, Switsky, Rotatori, & Vitkus (1982) have applied many of the previously described treatment procedures with mildly to moderately retarded children, adolescents, and adults. Persons undergoing treatment are trained to monitor daily weight and food intake, increase energy expenditure, reduce consumption rate, and reinforce their adherence to the program and progressive weight loss. Average weight loss over the course of the 14-week treatment period has been clinically significant, ranging from 3.7 to 10.2 pounds. The application of similar procedures to weight regulation in persons with Prader-Willi syndrome will be described in a subsequent section of the chapter.

INCREASING ACTIVITY LEVEL THROUGH EXERCISE

Application of learning theory principles to the modification of exercise participation has increased with growing interests in the fields of behavioral medicine and health psychology (Epstein & Wing, 1980; Martin & Dubbert, 1982). Behavioral approaches to exercise fall within three general target areas: (1) increasing energy expenditure as a component of weight reduction treatment programs, (2) enhancing physical fitness for cardiovascular risk reduction, and (3) teaching athletic performance to expand leisure-time activities.

The majority of studies in the behavioral literature on exercise have included some method of reinforcement as a primary treatment ingredient. The type of reinforcement delivery has been determined largely by the population under investigation and the goals of intervention. Since lack of maintenance to a regularly scheduled exercise regimen is a reoccurring problem (Martin, 1981), the effects of various reinforcement techniques to promote exercise adherence have been evaluated. In one study, Epstein, Wing, Thompson, and Griffin (1980) compared contingency contracting and lottery procedures with increase exercise attendance and physical fitness of 37 female college students. The students were required to run one or two miles per day during a 5-week aerobics exercise program. In the contingency contracting condition, each student deposited $5 preceding the study, portions of which were returned each week if they fulfilled predetermined attendance criteria. In the lottery condition, students who met attendance criteria each week received a lottery ticket. A drawing for either cash or a gift certificate was subsequently held at the study's conclusion. Overall, the results indicated that both contracting and lottery procedures were equally effective in significantly increasing exercise attendance when compared with a no-treatment control group.

In another application of contingency contracting, Wysocki, Hall, Iwata, and Riordan (1979) instructed college students to "give up" items of personal value. They subsequently permitted the students to earn back these items on a weekly basis if they accumulated a specified quantity of individually determined aerobics points and concurrently recorded the exercise performance of other participants. For seven of eight students, aerobic point earnings inceased dramatically over baseline levels with the introduction of the contracting procedures.

The previously described studies utilized participants who were interested in improving their physical fitness but otherwise represented a healthy, nonclinical population. What is the effectiveness of behavioral techniques for persons with identified problems? With obese children, increases in exercise participation and activity levels have been accomplished in several ways. For example, children have been reinforced on a point economy system for completion of programmed aerobic exercise or life-style activity changes such as walking instead of riding in a car and performing "on-the-spot" exercises while viewing television (Epstein, Wing, Koeske, Ossip, & Beck, 1982). Earned points were exchanged for special rewards. In another study, children were provided with reinforcers if they were "caught" engaging in specified active movements when a randomly scheduled signal was sounded (Epstein, Woodall, Goreczny, Wing, & Robertson, 1984). Among a developmentally disabled population, Allen and Iwata (1980) demonstrated that the performance of calisthenic-type exercises in mentally retarded adults could be increased by a simple manipulation in which access to a preferred activity (playing game) was made contingent upon completion of the exercises to criterion. The variety of reinforcers programmed, types of movement responses, and target subjects in these studies attest to the generality of behavioral intervention methods for promoting exercise participation.

Finally, individuals who fail to participate in a regular schedule of exercise may do so because the programmed activities are relatively monotonous and occur in isolation (e.g., jogging). The use of behavioral technology to teach athletic performance skills may be one way to overcome such difficulties (Allison & Ayllon, 1980). By training exercise habits in the context of competitive games, social support influences become operative, a variable that might lead to stronger response maintenance.

Decreasing Inappropriate Food-Related Behavior

Among the reported characteristics of Prader-Willi syndrome, several fall into the general category of inappropriate food-related behaviors (see Chapter 3, this volume). One that is frequently mentioned is eating unacceptable food products (e.g., Coplin, Hine, & Gormican, 1976) such as garbage and frozen food. Such behavior is frequently referred to as *pica*.

The vast majority of behavioral research on the treatment of pica has been conducted with severely to profoundly mentally retarded persons. Since the overriding clinical goal of such treatment is to produce rapid and complete suppression of this debilitating problem behavior, most intervention programs have utilized some form of response-contingent punishment. This point leads to an important caveat: the information related to individuals with profound retardation might not be appropriate for most individuals with Prader-Willi syndrome. Due to the type and frequency of pica that profoundly retarded individuals demonstrate, as well as their severe cognitive limitations, more intrusive techniques are necessary than would be for individuals with Prader-Willi syndrome. In severe cases among the Prader-Willi population, however, these approaches might have some merit.

Effective control of pica in mentally retarded individuals was reported in two studies using physical restraint procedures (Bucher, Reykdal, & Albin, 1976; Winton, & Singh, 1983). Contingent upon the display of pica or antecedents to the response, an attending adult grasped the individual's hands and held them by the sides of his/her body for several seconds. A visual screening procedure was employed by Singh and Winton (1984) to reduce pica in a 24-year-old, profoundly retarded woman. Each occurrence of pica resulted in removal of the object from her mouth followed by placement of a blindfold over her eyes for a 1 minute period. Two other important clinical findings emerged from this study. First, follow-up assessments conducted 1 to 6 months posttreatment revealed near-zero levels of pica despite the fact that the screening procedure was no longer operative. Secondly, during and following treatment, antecedents to pica, such as picking and handling inedible objects, decreased in frequency even though these responses were never directly consequated. As such, generalization of behavior change across responses and over time were associated with treatment in this case.

Overcorrection represents the most widely investigated technique for the behavior management of pica (Finney, Russo, & Cataldo, 1982; Foxx & Martin, 1975; Mulick, Barbour, Schroeder, & Rojahn, 1980). Characteristically, persons engaging in the behavior are required to perform repetitive cleansing of their mouths, hands, and/or physical environment. This procedure has two primary advantages over other treatment methods in that it is topographically related to the target problem and may provide for a hygienic effect.

Two types of nonaversive behavioral treatment have been used to reduce pica in children with lead poisoning. One approach incorporated a DRO procedure (Differential Reinforcement of Other Behavior; see Table 5.1) in which consumable reinforcers were presented to the children if they did not engage in pica behavior during specified time intervals (Finney et al., 1982). The second procedure consisted of discrimination training the entailed reinforcing the children for differentiating appropriately between edible and nonedible substances (Madden, Russo, & Cataldo, 1980). Although the design of nonaversive, reinforcement-based programs is always laudable, response reducton from such intervention is typically slow. Given the detrimental physical effects that can result from pica, such an approach must be considered cautiously.

In contrast to other behavior disorders, relatively few reports have appeared on the effective treatment of stealing. This may be due, in part, to the fact that the behavior is highly resistent to intervention given its immediate, self-reinforcing characteristics (Henderson, 1981). Also, it is often times difficult to observe the act of stealing and to impose treatment contingencies immediately upon detection.

Azrin and Wesolowski (1974) evaluated an overcorrection procedure to reduce food stealing of 34 institutionalized, severely to profoundly retarded adults. During a baseline phase, each resident who stole was required to return that item to its owner. Under this condition, an average of 120 stealing incidents occurred daily. During the overcorrection treatment phase, stolen items continued to be returned but, in addition, the thief was physically assisted through the process of obtaining an identical item and presenting it to the victim. Following four days of such treatment, stealing was virtually eliminated in all residents. The extremely rapid and complete suppression achieved in this study was most likely a function of the easily observed target behavior (e.g., snatching a food item out of another's hands) and the fact that the overcorrection consequence was applied immediately following each stealing incident.

DECREASING TANTRUMS AND AGGRESSION

There exists a voluminous literature concerning the behavior management of temper tantrums and aggressive disorders in children, adults, and the developmentally handicapped (Bornstein, Hamilton, & McFall, 1981; Mulick & Schroeder, 1980). Virtually every treatment strategy listed in Table 5.1 has been utilized with some degree of success in therapeutically controlling these problems. In this section, three sets of procedures will be reviewed: positive reinforcement, time-out, and social-skills training. These procedures have been selected for review because substantial research data exist attesting to their efficiency, and the fact that they are adaptable to a variety of applied settings.

The establishment of a positively reinforcing environment is essential in the design of any behavioral treatment program. This is a particularly relevant consideration in managing acting-out responses in the forms of tantrums and aggression. Because these behaviors are highly aversive to others, most individuals who display them are avoided, thereby experiencing limited, if any, positive interactions. This frequently results in an increase in disruptive responding, which produces further avoidance. Reinforcement procedures, therefore, must be programmed to interrupt this negative feedback loop.

The implementation of reinforcement can be accomplished in several ways. Using a DRO procedure, children can be presented with tangible reinforcers (e.g., consumable items, toys) when they fail to exhibit the problem behaviors during specified time periods (Luiselli, & Reisman, 1980; Luiselli & Slocumb, 1983). Similarly, tantrumous and aggressive behaviors might be reduced by providing a high density of reinforcement for compliance with adult-initiated instructions (Russo, Cataldo, & Cushing, 1981). This is possible because many management problems comprise a generalized class of noncompliant responding. Finally, reinforcement programs incorporating token economy procedures and contingency contracts have found extensive application in treating tantrumous and aggressive outbursts (Bornstein, et al., 1981). As always, the choice of a particular reinforcement method depends on the characteristics of the client, the severity of the presenting problem, the nature of the interpersonal/physical environment, and, most importantly, the identification of functionally reinforcing stimuli.

Many persons displaying tantrumous and aggressive behaviors remain unresponsive to positive reinforcement methods. When such a situation is encountered, a combined treatment approach can be developed by adding a response-contingent deceleration technique to an ongoing reinforcement strategy. One of the most effective procedures in this regard is the brief interruption in reinforcer availability through the imposition of a time-out contingency. When contemplating the implementation of time-out, practitioners should be cognizant of several concerns. First, use of time-out should not be considered if the behavior to be treated is reinforced by task avoidance and escape since this arrangement will only serve to maintain undesired responding. If application of contingent time-out is deemed appropriate, then thought must be given to which of several methods should be programmed. This choice is determined largely by variables in the treatment setting and response of the individual following institution of the time-out. For example, if the person being treated remains relatively nonagitated during the time-out period and does not receive attention from peers simultaneously, he/she can be required to sit away from the group setting while viewing ongoing activities, a procedure known as "contingent observation" (Porterfield, Herbert-Jackson, & Risley, 1976). Another form of nonexclusionary timeout consists of reinforcing an individual for wearing a prominently displayed stimulus such as a ribbon or badge and imposing time-out via removal of this discriminative cue (Foxx & Shapiro, 1978; Luiselli & Brown, 1987). In cases where the individual becomes more agitated or is able to elicit attention from others, time-out can be applied in an area removed from the center of activity such as a partitioned corner or a protective environment (Luiselli, 1987). Given situations where persistent and dangerous agitation occurs, seclusion time-out in an isolation room may be indicated (Drabman & Spitalnik, 1973; Luiselli, Myles, & Littman-Quinn, 1983). Whatever method is selected, it is desirable to program brief durations of time-out (e.g., 1–3 minutes) since excessively long periods can result in habituation and limit the individual's exposure to reinforcement for alternative, adaptive behaviors.

In some instances, individuals who engage in tantrumous and aggressive behaviors do so because they lack the interpersonal skills necessary to sustain reciprocal social interactions. Given the absence of such competencies, the violent and abusive behaviors serve to terminate difficult encounters and otherwise control the context of the social exchange. Teaching the requisite responses for appropriate interaction through social-skills training represents a viable therapeutic strategy in such cases (Borstein, Bellack, & Hersen, 1980; Frederiksen, Jenkins, Foy, & Eisler, 1976). The general format of this training begins by identifying the interpersonal situations that are creating problems for the individual. Then these situations are acted-out through role playing scenarios while the specific deficits in functioning are noted. These deficiencies might include avoiding sustained eye contact, speaking with limited voice volume, performing threatening physical gestures, or failing to make meaningful requests of the other partner. Once these deficits have been identified, the individual is then trained to perform the relevant skill. Such training is typically accomplished by having the individual observe modeled role-plays that depict proper use of the skill and then rehearse each skill accordingly. Feedback, coaching, and social reinforcement are provided by the therapist. Although in some instances such training may generalize to extra-therapy environments, it is usually advisable to establish contingencies that reinforce the individual's skill performance in "real world" settings. Generalization also can be promoted by actually conducting training in vivo.

Behavioral Treatment in Prader-Willi Syndrome

To date, a small body of research has emerged addressing the behavioral treatment of persons with Prader-Willi syndrome. Not surprisingly, the primary targets of this research have been the modification of eating habits and the reduction of body weight. In this section, the methodology and therapeutic outcome of these behavioral studies will be reviewed.

Altman, Bondy, and Hirsch (1978) reported one of the first behavioral studies with a Prader-Willi syndrome population. The participants were an 18-year-old, mildly retarded female weighing 224 pounds, and a 13-year-old, moderately retarded female weighing 121 pounds. Following a no-treatment baseline phase, each girl was reinforced for daily self-monitoring of caloric intake, body weight, and type/duration of exercise. Parents and care-givers also began recording incidents of food stealing. In a subsequent phase, reinforcement in the form of access to preferred activities was made contingent upon decreased caloric intake and body weight. In addition, any detected occurrences of food stealing were punished via public apologies, monetary fines, loss of privileges, and early bedtimes. Gradually, reinforcement was provided for weight loss alone and therapist contact with the participants was faded. Following a 1-year course of treatment, total weight losses of 65 and 30 pounds were achieved. The combination of reinforcement for caloric reduction and weight loss was shown to be the most effective treatment strategy. Weight losses continued to be observed for both participants at follow-up assessments of 3, 6, and 9 months.

Thompson, Kodluboy, and Heston (1980) also used a combination of procedures to treat a 22-year-old Prader-Willi female. The woman measured 4 feet 2 inches in height, weighed 179.25 pounds, and had a Stanford-Binet IQ of 75. Her initial treatment was conducted within a hospital setting and consisted of token economy points awarded for weight loss, response cost for weight gain, and social isolation following increases of .5 pounds or more each day. Throughout this hospitalization, consistent 1:1 monitoring of the patient was established. The remainder of treatment occurred in a private residence and day-activity-center. Because staff in these settings viewed the program as being punitive, it was withdrawn for a period of 2 months. However, no positive therapeutic effects were observed during this period and the point system was reinstated. Intervention was supplemented by twice weekly aversion relief therapy sessions in which electric shock in the presence of slides of high-calorie foods was applied, followed by shock termination in the presence of low-calorie food slides. Findings indicated that the most potent effects on weight resulted during a 5-month phase of 1:1 monitoring, immediate token reinforcement, and response cost (cumulative weight loss of 44 pounds). An additional 8 pounds were lost over a 3-month period of less structured environmental control. However, these reductions were evidenced after the woman gained 76 pounds in the absence of program contingencies. Thus, by the study's conclusion, her weight did not differ substantially from pretreatment levels.

Effective weight control was further demonstrated in a study by Marshall, Wallace, Elder, Burke, Oliver, and Blackmon (1981). The participants were four institutionalized residents with Prader-Willi syndrome, 20 to 26 years of age, with IQs in the 50 to 80 range. Weights and respective heights of each participant were 170 pounds (56"), 180 pounds (56"), 219 pounds (60"), and 235 pounds (58"). The treatment program consisted of: (1) training residents to consume one-half portions during meals, (2) requiring loss of meal portions and forfeited meals contingent upon specified problem behaviors (e.g., eating from others' plates, eating unauthorized foods between meals), and (3) granting grounds privileges for weekly weight loss of at least 1 pound and no more than two meal violations in the preceding week. Generalization prompting procedures also comprised the program and included the elimination of food monitoring, teaching proper selection of caloric food values, and establishing exercise participation. Over an 80-week treatment phase, the average weight loss per resident was an impressive 97.5 pounds. However, these results should be tempered by the fact that following discharge from the institutionalized treatment setting, three of the four participants gained back their preintervention weights. In all three cases, no program contingencies for feeding and weight control were operative in the posttreatment setting. This undoubtedly demonstrates the need for skills training in the natural environment.

Page, Finney, Parrish, and Iwata (1983) employed differential reinforcement procedures to eliminate food stealing in two Prader-Willi children within a controlled hospital setting. One child was an 8-year-old female with a WISC-R IQ of 75 who weighed 60 pounds; the second child was an 11-year-old male with a Stanford-Binet IQ of 46 weighing 135 pounds. The children were observed unobtrusively within three rooms in the hospital during regularly scheduled assessment sessions. Each room contained a variety of play items plus assorted edible snacks such as M&M candies, salted peanuts, and potato chips. Each instance of food stealing (placing a food item in contact with mouth) was recorded in a multiple baseline design across settings. Under baseline conditions, no contingencies were imposed for food stealing. The treatment program incorporated a DRO procedure in which the absence of stealing during a prescribed time interval was reinforced with tokens (poker chips). Whenever a child acquired 10 tokens at the conclusion of each session, he/she could exchange them for a low-calorie food item or a favorite toy. The interval began at 10 seconds and was increased gradually as the study progressed. As a result of this intervention, baseline rates of 6.1 to 8.4 steals per minute (child 1) and 1.3 to 2.6 steals per minute (child 2) were reduced immediately to near-zero levels. During subsequent follow-up assessments within the hospital, decreased rates of stealing were maintained. At these follow-up visits, however, both children had gained weight, indicating that food stealing likely continued within their natural environments. Again, *without deliberate programming in extratherapy settings*, it is unlikely that the positive effects achieved in a controlled therapeutic milieu will be sustained.

Finally, the findings reported by Page et al. (1983) were replicated in a study of a 28-year-old woman with Prader-Willi syndrome by Page, Stanley, Richman, Deal, and Iwata (1983). The woman had a WAIS IQ of 55, was 56 inches in height, and weighed 253 pounds. In addition to reducing food stealing, a weight reduction program also was developed. Treatment was initially implemented during an in-patient hospitalization and featured token reinforcement for progressive weight loss and participation in a specially designed exercise regimen. Loss of tokens was made cotingent upon detected food thefts. Following the hospitalization, treatment contingencies were extended to community group-home and, subsequently, apartment-living arrangement. Over a 2-year period, a total of 81 pounds was lost, with reductions maintained within the posthospitalization environments.

Summary

This chapter has documented the effective use of behavior therapy for treating persons with Prader-Willi syndrome. A variety of procedures has been shown to produce meaningful changes in adaptive skills, management problems, and physical well-being. Clearly, behavioral methods have much to offer in designing comprehensive care programs for the individual with Prader-Willi syndrome. The continued success of such programming will depend upon careful attention to several critical issues. Therapeutic changes in behavior, for example, tend to be highly situation-specific. That is, control over responding typically occurs for behaviors that are explicitly treated, within settings where treatment is ongoing, and in the presence of those who apply program contingencies. As evident in many of the studies reviewed previously, generalized changes arc quite clearly the exception rather than the rule. Teaching a child with Prader-Willi syndromc not to steal in a hospital or clinic setting is no indication that he/she will inhibit stealing inside the home (Page et al., 1983). Similarly, effective weight loss achieved during treatment is unlikely to be supported following an abrupt discontinuation of programming (Marshall et al., 1981).

Generalizing behavior change during treatment or maintaining therapy gains once intervention is discontinued must be viewed as an active process. Thus, practitioners and clinicians should be prepared to "program out" the differences between treated and nontreated behaviors and settings as a means to establish generalization and maintenance (Marholin, Sigel, & Phillips, 1976; Stokes, & Baer, 1977). The following represent possible facilitative strategies in this regard: (1) introducing treatment contingencies into all relevant settings, (2) having treatment applied by multiple change-agents, (3) establishing social stimuli as functional reinforcers, (4) training clients in self-management, (5) developing behaviors that are incompatible with the target problems, (6) programming types of delays in reinforcement delivery that are comparable with those in extra-therapy settings, and (7) introducing discriminative cues into treatment that have a high probability of occurring in the posttreatment environment.

Social validity refers to the acceptance of a clinical intervention and resulting therapeutic change by the recipients of therapy, treatment mediators, and community members at large (Wolf, 1979). This concern with "consumer satisfaction" has been an expanding interest of many behavior therapists and researchers (Bornstein & Rychtarik, 1983; McMahon & Forehand, 1983). Evaluating the acceptability of treatment mehtods and outcomes is an essential step in designing and packaging therapy programs. For example, an effective behavior-change methodology will find limited use if practitioners consistently view it in a negative light. Similarly, a client will reluctantly carry out a treatment plan that is judged to be harsh, cumbersome, and the like. A concern for the legal and ethical safeguards of clients also underscores the importance of social validity measurement in behavior therapy as well as other forms of psychological treatment.

In most of the studies in this chapter, individuals such as parents, teachers, therapy aides, and institutional staff were responsible for implementing treatment. Ensuring that treatment programs are administered properly by these practitioners is a crucial element for clinical success. Although it has been demonstrated that paraprofessionals can be taught to apply behavioral methods (Graziano & Katz, 1982), fewer research studies have compared the relative effectiveness of different instructional training formats. For instance, how differentially effective is training conducted on an individual versus group basis? Can various audio-visual materials enhance instruction? What types of self-help manuals are most useful? Answers to these and similar questions will lead to improvements in our instructional technology. At the same time, continued efforts must be directed at discovering methods that will motivate change-agents to implement procedures consistently and as formulated. How many therapists and clinicians have successfully trained parents to apply an intervention program only to find that the program is not carried out once training is terminated? On many occasions, ineffective therapy results not as a function of a poorly conceived plan but rather, inconsistent and improper implementation. This is an important consideration since the maladaptive behavior exhibited by individuals with Prader-Willi syndrome are persistent throughout life.

In conclusion, behavior analysis and therapy represents a useful methodology for treating persons with Prader-Willi syndrome. The strengths of a behavioral orientation are its commitment to functional assessment, empirical validation, and close scrutiny of how interpersonal variables affect responding. Perhaps the most meaningful implication to be gleaned from this review is that a behavioral approach is multipurposeful in function, can be integrated constructively with other therapeutic disciplines, and used in a variety of settings. Given the many medical, educational, and psychological dictates of the individual with Prader-Willi syndrome, the importance of a multidisciplinary treatment approach cannot be overemphasized.

REFERENCES

Allen, L. D., & Iwata, B. A. (1980). Reinforcing exercise maintenance using high-rate activities. *Behavior Modification, 4,* 337–354.

Allison, M. G., & Ayllon, T. (1980). Behavioral coaching in the development of skills in football, gymnastics, and tennis. *Journal of Applied Behavior Analysis, 13,* 297–314.

Altman, K., Bondy, A., & Hirsch, G. (1978). Behavioral treatment of obesity in patients with Prader-Willi syndrome. *Journal of Behavioral Medicine, 1,* 403–412.

Azrin, N. H., & Wesolowski, M. D. (1974). Theft reversal: An overcorrection procedure for eliminating stealing by retarded persons. *Journal of Applied Behavior Analysis, 7,* 577–581.

Bornstein, M., Bellack, A. S., & Hersen, M. (1980). Social skills training for highly aggressive children: Treatment in an inpatient psychiatric setting. *Behavior Modification, 4,* 173–186.

Bornstein, P. H., Hamilton, S. B., & McFall, M. E. (1981). Modification of adult aggression: A critical review of theory, research, and practice. In M. Hersen, R. M. Eisler & P. M. Miller (Eds.), *Progress in behavior modification, volume 12* (pp. 299–350). New York: Academic Press.

Bornstein, P. H., & Rychtarik, R. G. (1983). Consumer satisfaction in adult behavior therapy: Procedures, problems, and future perspectives. *Behavior Therapy, 14,* 191–208.

Brownell, K. D. (1982). Obesity: Understanding and treating a serious, prevalent, and refractory disorder. *Journal of Consulting and Clinical Psychology, 50,* 820–840.

Bucher, B. B., Reykdal, B., & Albin, J. (1976). Brief restraint to control pica in retarded children. *Journal of Behavior Therapy and Experimental Psychiatry, 7,* 137–140.

Carr, E. G., Newsom, C. D., & Binkoff, J. A. (1980). Escape as a factor in the aggressive behavior of two retarded children. *Journal of Applied Behavior Analysis, 13,* 101–117.

Coplin, S. S., Hine, J., & Gormican, A. (1976). Out-patient dietary management in the Prader-Willi syndrome. *Journal of the American Dietetic Association, 68,* 330–334.

Coates, T. J., & Thoresen, C. E. (1981). Behavior and weight changes in three obese adolescents. *Behavior Therapy, 12,* 383–399.

Drabman, R. S., Cordua, G. D., Hammer, D., Jarvie, G. J., & Horton, W. (1979). Developmental trends in eating rates of normal and overwieght preschool children. *Child Development, 50,* 211–216.

Drabman, R. S., Hammer, D., & Jarvie, G. J. (1977). Eating styles of obese and non-obese black and white children in a naturalistic setting. *Addictive Behaviors, 2,* 83–86.

Drabman, R. S., & Spitalnik, R. (1973). Social isolation as a punishment procedure: A controlled study. *Journal of Experimental Child Psychology, 16,* 236–249.

Epstein, L. H., Masek, B. J., & Marshall, W. R. (1978). A nutritionally-based school programs for control of eating in obese children. *Behavior Therapy, 9,* 766–778.

Epstein, L. H., Parker, L., McCoy, J. F., & McGee, G. (1976). Descriptive analysis of eating regulations in obese and nonobese children. *Journal of Applied Behavior Analysis, 7,* 402–416.

Epstein, L. H., & Wing, R. R. (1980). Behavioral approaches to exercise habits and athletic performance. In J. Ferguson & C. B. Taylor (Eds.), *Advances in behavioral medicine, 1,* Holliswood, NY: Spectrum.

Epstein, L. H., Wing, R. R., Koeske, R., Ossip, D. J., & Beck, S. (1982). A comparison of life-style change and programmed aerobic exercise on weight and fitness changes in obese children. *Behavior Therapy, 13,* 651–665.

Epstein, L. H., Wing, R. R., Thompson, J. K., & Griffin, W. (1980). Attendance and fitness in aerobics exercise. *Behavior Modification, 4,* 465–479.

Epstein, L. H., Woodall, K., Goreczny, A. J., Wing, R. R., & Robertson, R. J. (1984). The modification of activity patterns and energy expenditure in obese young girls. *Behavior Therapy, 15,* 101–108.

Finney, J. W., Russo, D. C., & Cataldo, M. F. (1982). Reduction of pica in young children with lead poisoning. *Journal of Pediatric Psychology, 7,* 197–207.

Foxx, R., Switsky, H., Rotatori, A., & Vitkus, P. (1982). Successful weight loss techniques with mentally retarded children and youth. *Exceptional Children, 49,* 238–244.

Foxx, R. M., & Martin, E. D. (1975). Treatment of scavenging behavior (copraphagy and pica) by overcorrection. *Behavior Research and Therapy, 13,* 153–162.

Foxx, R. M., & Shapiro, S. T. (1978). The time-out ribbon: A nonexclusionary time-out procedure. *Journal of Applied Behavior Analysis, 11,* 125–136.

Frederiksen, L. W., Jenkins, J. O., Foy, D. W., & Eisler, R. M. (1976). Social skills training in the modification of abusive verbal outbursts in adults. *Journal of Applied Behavior Analysis, 9,* 117–125.

Graziano, A. M., & Katz, J. N. (1982). Training paraprofessionals. In A. A. Bellack, M. Hersen, & A. E. Kazdin (Eds.), *International handbook of behavior modification and therapy* (pp. 207–229). New York: Plenum Press.

Henderson, J. Q. (1981). A behavioral approach to stealing: A proposal for treatment based on ten cases. *Journal of Behavior Therapy and Experimental Psychiatry, 12,* 231–236.

Hersen, M., & Barlow, D. H. (1984). *Single case experimental designs: Strategies for studying behavior change.* New York: Pergamon Press.

Hersen, M., & Bellack, A. S. (Eds.). (1978). *Behavior therapy in the psychiatric setting.* Baltimore, MD: Williams and Wilkins.

Hersen, M., & Bellack, A. S. (1981). *Behavioral assessment.* New York: Pergamon Press.

Kanner, L. (1957). *Child psychiatry.* Springfield, IL: Charles C. Thomas.

Kazdin, A. E. (1982a). History of behavior modification. In A. A. Bellack, M. Hersen, & A. E. Kazdin (Eds.), *International handbook of behavior modification and therapy.* (pp. 3–32). New York: Plenum Press.

Kazdin, A. E. (1982b). *Single case research designs: Methods for clinical and applied settings.* New York: Oxford.

Keane, T. M., Geller, S. E., & Scheirer, C. J. (1981). A parametric investigation of eating styles in obese and nonobese children. *Behavior Therapy, 12,* 280–286.

Luiselli, J. D. (1987). Behavioral medicine research and treatment in developmental disabilities. In R. Barrett & J. L. Matson (Eds.), *Advances in developmental disorders.* (pp. 1–39). Greenwich, CT: JAI Press.

Luiselli, J. K. (1987). *Behavior management in a deaf-blind youth using response interruption and protective environment time-out.* Manuscript submitted for publication.

Luiselli, J. K., & Brown, C. A. (1987). *Combining reinforcement and nonexclusionary time-out procedures in a residential treatment program for aggressive, mentally retarded adults.* Manuscript submitted for publication.

Luiselli, J. K., Myles, E., & Littman-Quinn, J. (1983). Analysis of a reinforcement/time-out treatment package to control severe aggressive and destructive behaviors in a multihandicapped, rubella child. *Applied Research in Mental Retardation, 4,* 65–78.

Luiselli, J. K., & Reisman, J. (1980). Some variations in the use of differential reinforcement procedures with mentally retarded children in specialized treatment settings. *Applied Research in Mental Retardation, 1,* 277–288.

Luiselli, J. K., & Slocumb, P. R. (1983). Management of multiple aggressive behaviors by differential reinforcement. *Journal of Behavior Therapy and Experimental Psychiatry, 14,* 343–347.

Lutzker, J. R., Martin, J. A., & Rice, J. M. (1981). Behavior therapy in rehabilitation. In M. Hersen, R.M. Eisler, & P.M. Miller (Eds.), *Progress in behavior modification.* (Vol. 12, pp. 171–226). New York: Academic Press.

Madden, N. A., Russo, D. C., & Cataldo, M. F. (1980). Behavioral treatment of pica in children with lead poisoning. *Child Behavior Therapy, 2,* 67–81.

Mahoney, M. J. (1974). *Cognition and behavior modification.* Cambridge, MA: Ballinger.

Marholin II, D., Siegel, L. J., & Phillips, D. (1976). Treatment and transfer: A search for empirical procedures. In M. Hersen, R. M. Eisler, & P. M. Miller (Eds.), *Progress in behavioral modification.* (Vol. 3, pp. 293–342). New York: Academic Press.

Marshall, B. D., Wallace, C. J., Elder, J., Burke, K., Oliver, T., & Blackmon, R. (1981). A behavioral approach to treatment of Prader-Willi syndrome. In W. A. Holm, S. J. Sulzbacher, & P. L. Pipes (Eds.), *Prader-Willi syndrome.* Baltimore, MD: University Park Press.

Martin, J. E. (1981). Exercise management: Shaping and maintaining physical fitness. *Behavioral Medicine Advances, 4,* 3–5.

Martin, J. E., & Dubbert, P. M. (1982). Exercise applications and promotion in behavioral medicine: Current status and future directions. *Journal of Consulting and Clinical Psychology, 50,* 1004–1017.

Masek, B. J., Epstein, L. H., & Russo, D. C. (1981). Behavioral perspectives in preventive medicine. In S. M. Turner, K. S. Calhoun, & H. E. Adams (Eds.), *Handbook of clinical behavior therapy.* (pp. 475–499). New York: Wiley.

McMahon, R. J., & Forehand, R. L. (1983). Consumer satisfaction in behavioral treatment in children: Types, issues, and recommendations. *Behavior Therapy, 14,* 209-225.

Morris, R. J., & Brown, K. (1983). Legal issues in behavior modification with the mentally retarded. In J. L. Matson & F. Andrasik (Eds.), *Treatment issues and innovations in mental retardation.* (pp. 61-96). New York: Plenum Press.

Mulick, J. A., Barbour, R., Schroeder, S. R., & Rojahn, J. (1980). Overcorrection of pica in two profoundly retarded adults: Analysis of setting events, stimulus, and response generalization. *Applied Research in Mental Retardation, 1,* 241-252.

Mulick, J. A., & Schroeder, S. R. (1980). Research relating to management of antisocial behavior in mentally retarded persons. *The Psychological Record, 30,* 397-417.

Page, T. J., Finney, J. W., Parrish, J. M., & Iwata, B. A. (1983). Assessment and reduction of food stealing in Prader-Willi children. *Applied Research in Mental Retardation, 4,* 219-228.

Page, T. J., Stanley, A. E., Richman, G. S., Deal, R. M., & Iwata, B. A. (1983). Reduction of food theft and long-term maintenance of weight loss in a Prader-Willi adult. *Journal of Behavior Therapy and Experimental Psychiatry, 14,* 261-268.

Porterfield, J. K., Herbert-Jackson, E., & Risley, T. R. (1976). Contingent observation: An effective and acceptable procedure for reducing disruptive behavior of young children in a group setting. *Journal of Applied Behavior Analysis, 9,* 55-64.

Russo, D. C., Cataldo, M. F., & Cushing, P. J. (1981). Compliance training and behavioral covariation in the treatment of multiple behavior problems. *Journal of Applied Behavior Analysis, 14,* 209-222.

Singh, N. N., & Winton, A. S. W. (1984). Effects of a screening procedure on pica and collateral behaviors. *Journal of Behavior Therapy and Experimental Psychiatry, 15,* 59-65.

Skinner, B. F. (1953). *Science and human behavior.* New York: MacMillan.

Stokes, T. F., & Baer, D. M. (1977). An implicit technology of generalization. *Journal of Applied Behavior Analysis, 10,* 349-367.

Stunkard, A. J. (1982). Obesity. In A. S. Bellack, M. Hersen, & A. E. Kazdin (Eds.), *International handbook of behavior modification and therapy.* (pp. 535-573). New York: Plenum Press.

Thompson, T., Kodluboy, S., & Heston, L. (1980). Behavioral treatment of obesity in Prader-Willi syndrome. *Behavior Therapy, 11,* 588-593.

Varni, J. W. (1983). *Clinical behavioral pediatrics.* New York: Pergamon Press.

Winton, A. S. W., & Singh, N. N. (1983). Suppression of pica using brief-duration physical restraint. *Journal of Mental Deficiency Research, 27,* 93-103.

Wetherby, B., & Baumeister, A. A. (1981). Mental retardation. In S. M. Turner, C. S. Calhoun, & H. E. Adams (Eds.), *Handbook of clinical behavior therapy.* (pp. 635-664). New York: Wiley.

Wolf, M. M. (1979). Social validity: The case for subjective measurement of how applied behavior analysis is finding its heart. *Journal of Applied Behavior Analysis, 11,* 203-214.

Wysocki, T., Hall, G., Iwata, B. A., & Riordan, M. (1979). Behavioral management of exercise: Contracting for aerobics points. *Journal of Applied Behavior Analysis, 12,* 55-64.

6
Surgical Considerations in Prader-Willi Syndrome

CHARLES W. WAGNER

Surgical involvement for individuals with Prader-Willi syndrome, although important, is usually for secondary reasons. In general, nonsurgical aggressive and/or conservative manuevers are tried before surgical procedures are considered. Fortunately, these nonsurgical procedures usually succeed, at least to a better level of satisfaction than surgery is likely to offer; these treatments typically are safer and have fewer complications. In general, pediatric surgeons are consulted for weight control, gonadal surgery, spinal curve stabilization, and occasionally cosmetic reconstruction. Discussion of each of these areas follows.

Characterization of Prader-Willi syndrome has been that of the HHHO syndrome (hypogonadism, hypotonia, hypomentia, and obesity; Zellweger & Schneider, 1968). Obesity typically has its onset between the ages of 6 months and 6 years. The average time is around 2 years of age and, if uncontrolled, weight gain will continue throughout childhood, puberty, and adulthood. It has been suggested that children with Prader-Willi syndrome appear to have a persistent hunger with little sense of satiety. It is also reported that they constantly ask for food and will forage in any location for both appropriate and inappropriate substances. The hyperphagia is a major predisposing factor in the obesity of these patients (Bray, Dahms, Swerdloff, Fiser, Atkinson, & Carrel, 1983; Laurance, Brito, & Wilkinson, 1981; Nelson, Huse, Holman, Kimbrogh, Wahner, Callaway, & Hayles, 1981). Also, some studies have shown a decreased caloric requirement in Prader-Willi individuals. Pipes (1981) documented weight maintenance in patients with Prader-Willi syndrome with a dietary intake of 10 to 11 kcal/cm of height. Children without the syndrome required between 12 and 22 kcal/cm of height for their maintenance of weight.

The problems of obesity and the need for attempts to control weight are critical. Individuals with Prader-Willi syndrome develop non-insulin-dependent diabetes, which has been directly related to weight gain; subsequently, control of the diabetes has resulted in weight loss (Bistrian, Blackburn, & Stanbury, 1977; Hall & Smith, 1972; Laurance, Brito, & Wilkinson, 1981). Other side effects are the development of the Pickwickian syndrome of hypercapnia, hypoxia, and right-sided heart failure (Cassidy, 1984). The cause of the symptoms is related to the compression and decreased expansion of the lungs due to the fat mass. This starts the vicious cycle of carbon dioxide retention, acidosis, constriction of pulmonary arterioles, and pulmonary hypertension. There is also a predilection for pulmonary embolism in this situation (Rochester & Enson, 1974).

Because of the extreme obesity, a shortened life expectancy is characteristic of individuals with Prader-Willi syndrome (Soper, Mason, Printen, & Zellweger, 1981) and control of obesity would appear to have important benefits. Also, while the psychological and social impact of the morbid obesity in Prader-Willi syndrome is not clear, it is entirely possible that it does have a negative effect on their self-image. The improved self-image of patients with Prader-Willi via weight reduction has been the experience of those at the University of Connecticut Prader-Willi syndrome clinic (Cassidy, 1981).

Surgery for Obesity Control

Obesity control is one area for which surgical techniques may be of aid to patients with Prader-Willi syndrome. While dietary control is always the first step in this population, the long-term outcome may be less than satisfactory. As the child grows and becomes more independent, strict control of his dietary intake becomes less and less possible. To address these problems, surgical procedures have been developed for the control of morbid obesity after failure or relapse with dietary control has occurred.

While there are a number of different operations available, they essentially can be divided into two general categories that address the basis of the obesity found in Prader-Willi syndrome. The procedures are either the small bowel (jejunoileal) bypass or the gastric bypass/gastroplasty (gastric stapling). The benefit and risks of each procedure will be discussed separately.

Small bowel or jejunoileal bypass has long been popularized for weight control. It works by way of bypassing up to 90% of the small intestine. Weight loss then occurs because of decreased absorption of fats and carbohydrates (Randolph, Weintraub, & Rigg, 1974) thereby decreasing the caloric intake. The patient is not required to change either his eating habits or diet in order to lose weight. Most of the surgical experience for weight reductions has been with adults without Prader-Willi syndrome who are morbidly obese, but there are reported cases in the adolescent age-group (White, Cheek, & Haller, 1974) and for those with Prader-Willi syndrome (Randolph, Weintraub, & Rigg, 1974). Initially weight loss and stabilization are excellent, although there have been reports of significant long-term problems. In jejunoileal bypass, diarrhea is common with the occurrence of severe dehydration and electrolyte imbalance. Protein malnutrition, cirrhosis, renal calculi, cholelithiasis, polyarthritis, pancreatitis, and psychiatric problems have also been documented in any range from 5 to 40% of patients (Alden, 1977; Kuldau & Rand, 1980; Organ, Cegielski, Grabner, Keig, & Saporta, 1980; Scott, 1980). Experimentally, Grosfeld, Cooney, Csicsko, and Madura (1976) demonstrated adverse effects of the jejunoileal bypass in rats. Interestingly, the long-term follow up of adolescents with and without Prader-Willi syndrome, while few in number, has not demonstrated a high incidence of side effects. Similarly, the procedures did not appear to affect growth and development in this younger group.

The gastric bypass and, more recently, gastroplasty were introduced to overcome the severe complications of the jejunoileal bypass. The gastric bypass involves the formation of a measured stomach pouch (usually 50 cc) and a newly created gastroenterostomy for emptying of food (Hartford, 1984; Mason, 1982). The gastroplasty involves the formation of a measured volume stomach compartment, although the food is emptied directly into the stomach thereby requiring no enterostomy. The stomach is partitioned with the size of the outlet determining the rate of emptying (Smith, 1981). While there are further nuances for each procedure, the end result of these procedures is the decreased intake of food because of early satiety or vomiting. Results of the operations have been good in obese individuals with and without Prader-Willi syndrome (Anderson, Soper, & Scott, 1980). However, the weight loss has not been as large as that using the small bowel bypass, and stabilization occurs at about 1 year. There also has been reported a rebounding or regaining of the lost weight. In other studies, however (non-Prader-Willi patients), better results have been obtained (Smith, Fricke, & Graney, 1983). The most striking finding is the absence of the significant side effects noted in the jejunoileal bypass (Ackerman, 1982; Flickenger, Pories, Meelheim, Sinar, Blose, & Thomas, 1984; Kuldau & Rand, 1980; Rucker, Horstmann, Schneider, Varco, & Buchwald, 1982; Smith, 1981). The problems associated with the gastric procedures include the need for revision of the outlet. Anderson et al. (1980) reported 11 cases in which six patients required later revisions. Leaks from the gastroenterostomy and splenic injury also are reported and may add to the early and late morbidity (Flickenger, et.al., 1984). Furthermore, since the results of the surgery rely on early satiety and the eating habits of individuals with Prader-Willi syndrome are by nature unpredictable, the end result may be less than satisfactory. In essence, the individual may outeat (by small constant feeds) his operation. Fonkalsrud and Bray (1981) reported an attempt at controlling the obesity in Prader-Willi syndrome by performing a truncal vagotomy. The mechanism of action of this method is the development of early satiety by gastric stasis, thereby curbing the appetite. The patient initially had an excellent response but soon gained back nearly 70% of his weight loss. It was soon discovered that the individual had been eating multiple small feedings such that he increased his caloric intake. Indeed, studies indicate that close follow up is needed in the obese patient with a gastric bypass for the best results. Patients who missed appointments had significantly less weight reduction than those who maintained the prescribed visits. Another potential problem with the gastric procedure is that good dental hygiene is necessary so that nutrition can be maintained. Food ingested must undergo good mastication so that it can pass out of the stomach. Dental caries are common (44%) and are related to poor hygiene and frequent meals (Zellweger & Schneider, 1968). Enamelyplasia was noted in 12% of patients in another series (Nelson, et. al., 1981).

In summary, surgical control of the obesity of individuals with Prader-Willi syndrome can be obtained, although as with any operation, the successful end result must not be gained at the cost of serious unwanted complications. Both the jejunoileal bypass and the gastric bypass/gastroplasty have proven to be successful (Kuldau & Rand, 1980). The jejunoileal bypass has worked with Prader-Willi patients and has shown constant results in the adolescent population. Severe side effects in the adult population, however, should make one careful about its application. The gastric procedures are effective but carry with them the need for possible reoperation for revision. Some of the perioperative complications are severe and long-standing, and there is the possibility of long-term failure for individuals with Prader-Willi syndrome.

Cosmetic Surgery

The distribution of fat in Prader-Willi syndrome is most prominent over the trunk, buttocks, and thighs. Sparing occurs in the hands, feet, and distal extremities. If weight reduction occurs, the process reverses itself and the end fat distribution is still central in nature. So while the shoulder, face, neck, and extremities are thin, the trunk, buttocks, and thighs remain large and redundant.

In adolescent obese patients, initially it was felt that the redundant skin would remold, although this is rarely the case (Anderson et al., 1980; White, et al., 1974). Therefore, panniculectomies, subcutaneous mastectomies, thigh reduction, buttock reduction, and body sculpturing techniques can be considered for these patients once weight stabilization has occurred. Reports are few and follow up not adequate in the Prader-Willi patients for firm recommendations. Another consideration is the use of costoplasty. This involves resection and remolding of the ribs in patients who have undergone fixation of their scoliosis (Gurd & Thompson, 1981). The surgery is used to correct rib prominence in convexity rib depression in concavity, and anterior chest asymmetry. This has been used in non-Prader-Willi individuals with good success.

Scoliosis Surgery

Scoliosis is common in the Prader-Willi population. Holm and Laurnen (1981) reported that of the 37 Prader-Willi patients studied by skeletal films, 32 had a greater than 10° curvature, while the normal population has a 1 to 2% incidence of the same measurement. The scoliosis is similar to idiopathic scoliosis and is not related to obesity. However, obesity may affect the ease on difficulty of management whether with bracing or by surgery.

Patients should be followed for their scoliosis (Carr, Moe, Winter, & Lonstein, 1980). Progression may occur slowly, rapidly, or not at all. Bracing is recommended for curvatures that are progressive and near 20°. Bracing functions stop the worsening of their curvature. Bracing will not correct the curvature to normal and must be used until skeletal maturity is achieved. This treatment requires cooperation of the patient, which is sometimes difficult.

Curvatures greater than 45° should be surgically stabilized (Laurnen, 1981). This includes the use of Harrington rods and spinal fusion. Nontreatment of this severe scoliosis can lead to ventilation problems and cardiopulmonary dysfunction. This occurs in a group already susceptible to these problems (Orenstein et al., 1980). As is the case with bracing, cooperation is necessary as the patient is placed in a protective cast until fusion becomes solid.

Gonadal and Genitalia Surgery

Hypogonadism as well as undescended testicles are present in the majority of males with Prader-Willi syndrome. Half of all males with Prader-Willi Syndrome have bilateral undescended testes, and half of those remaining have unilateral undescended testes. The descent with gonadotropin has been good in most cases and certainly should be tried first. However, biopsies of the testes in other series have shown poor or absent spermatogonia, but moderate sertoli cell appearance (Uehling, 1980; Wannarachue, Ruvalcaba, & Kelly, 1975). Most males with Prader-Willi syndrome have low circulating testosterone and, in fact, respond rather poorly to therapy with human choriogonadotropins (Garty, Shuper, Mimouni, Varsano, & Kauli, 1982; Hamilton, Scully, & Kliman, 1972). Females with Prader-Willi syndrome have near normal rises in luteinizing hormone and follicle-stimulating hormone following treatment with 200 mg/day oral clomiphene (McGuffin & Rogol, 1975).

Surgery in male patients with Prader-Willi syndrome for undescended testes should follow the same general guidelines as in other males with undescended testes (Uehling, 1980). In bilateral cases, serum testosterone levels should be measured before and after stimulation. Ultrasound may be used in an attempt to localize any nonpalpable testes. Surgical repair as an out-patient at age 2 to 4 years is recommended. This age range allows for some natural descent, while simultaneously offering a safe age for surgery and minimizing the psychological trauma related to gonadal surgery in a male. Surgery first is performed on the side expected to be less complicated; if it takes less than 45 minutes and the testicle is not under too much tension, then the second side also is explored if it is undescended. However, if the first side is difficult in any way, then the second side is delayed for 3 to 6 months for safety. This reduces the risk of destruction of both of the testes simultaneously. The Dartos pouch reconstruction technique is recommended, and the results for maintaining scrotal position should be as satisfactory as it is in the general population of males. It is important for the family to be apprised of the overall poor gonadal function in children with Prader-Willi syndrome so that they fully understand the consequences of this surgery.

Hypogonadism is seen in a significant number of both males and females with Prader-Willi syndrome. Surgery to alter the appearance of the genitalia alone should be avoided unless absolutely necessary (Holm, 1981). The results are not impressive, and the need for such anatomic repair is probably very low. Some of the males that have a small penis have responded to twice daily applications of topical testosterone cream. Occasionally, iron testosterone also has had some success in increasing the size of the penis. As with other forms of abnormally small male genitalia, reconstruction to near normal size is not really possible.

The females with Prader-Willi syndrome tend to have a small clitoris as well as undeveloped labia. These problems may not be noticed in the newborn period, however, and usually are observed somewhat later in life. Surgical repair of these problems is rarely necessary, but can be done.

Surgery for Miscellaneous Problems

Several miscellaneous problems occasionally requiring surgical subspecialists have been reported in children with Prader-Willi syndrome. These problems indicate the importance of having the pediatric surgeon fully involved with children with Prader-Willi syndrome as they are being watched by other primary care-givers. Although this has not been the present author's personal experience, some of the hypotonic infants require the placement of either gastrostomy tubes or hyperalimentation lines to prevent poor feeding in the neonatal period. Rarely, gastric perforation has been reported in children with Prader-Willi syndrome secondary to massive ingestion of foods. The treatment of this is obviously surgical and follows standard guidelines for gastric perforation. Children with Prader-Willi syndrome also have been reported to have an increased incidence of strabismus (Hall & Smith, 1972). Repair by pediatric ophthalmologists should be done with the standard guidelines for other children with similar problems.

Anesthetic Considerations in Children with Prader-Willi Syndrome

Consideration of the anesthetic management in Prader-Willi syndrome can be approached from a technical and metabolic viewpoint. These are all related to the identifiable abnormalities within the syndrome.

Technically, these patients have dental problems, which make their teeth fragile (Palmer & Atleer, 1976). Because of this, care must be exercised at the time of intubation. Individuals with Prader-Willi syndrome also have high arched palates and micrognathia causing intubation difficulties (Yamashita, Koishi, Yamaya, Tsubo, Matube, & Oyama, 1983). Hypotonia may cause the cough reflex to be weak and obesity may make adequate ventilation difficult. Scoliosis also decreases the ability to ventilate the child who is asleep.

Metabolic derangements include diabetic abnormalities in the older obese child (Palmer & Atlee, 1976; Yamashita, Koishi, Yamaya, Tsubo, Matube, & Oyama, 1983). These problems can be managed somewhat easier for these children than for a true insulin-dependent diabetic. Both younger and older children have shown thermal instability with either hypothermia or hyperthermia as the end result. The hyperthermia, however, does not appear to be related to the reported malignant hyperthermia syndrome and both hypothermia and hyperthermia can be treated by mechanical means (i.e., cooling/warming blanket). There appears to be no benefit in using Dantrolene. Cardiac arrhythmias have been reported, but cannot be related to specific conditions of the child with Prader-Willi syndrome. Convulsions occur with this syndrome, and epileptogenic agents are used with extreme care.

In spite of hypotonia, anesthetic management can be done with muscle relaxants (short-acting) without reported problems. Halothane appears to be the agent of choice because of the absence of hyperglycemic effects, easy controllability, nonepileptogenic side effects, and easy respiratory control. Although cardiac arrhythmias are reported, careful use of halothane appears to have no increased incidence of problems for children with Prader-Willi syndrome.

Summary

Surgical intervention for individuals with Prader-Willi syndrome is almost exclusively secondary to other intervention approaches. In general, jejunoileal bypass or gastric-stapling procedures are sometimes used for obesity control with this population. Cosmetic surgery such as thigh and buttock reductions also has been attempted. Surgical corrections for problems such as scoliosis and hypogonadism also are sometimes conducted. In general, surgical procedures follow the same guidelines as those for individuals without Prader-Willi syndrome who present with similar characteristics (e.g., extreme obesity). A number of considerations regarding anesthesia of individuals with Prader-Willi syndrome must be addressed. These include caution at the time of intubation and awareness of potential thermal instability of the patient.

REFERENCES

Ackerman, N. (1982). Changes in serum cholesterol and triglyceride level after jejunoileal and gastric bypasses in morbidly obese patients. *Surgery, Gynecology, and Obstetrics, 154,* 1–7.

Alden, J. (1977). Gastric and jejunoileal bypass: A comparison in the treatment of morbid obesity. *Archives of Surgery, 112,* 799–806.

Anderson, A., Soper, R., & Scott, D. (1980). Gastric bypass for morbid obesity in children and adolescents. *Journal of Pediatric Surgery, 15,* 876–881.

Bistrian, B., Blackburn, G., & Stanbury, J. (1977). Metabolic aspects of protein-sparing modified fast in the dietary management of Prader-Willi obesity. *New England Journal of Medicine, 296,* 774–779.

Bray, G., Dahms, W., Swerdloff, R., Fiser, R., Atkinson, R., & Carrel, R. (1983). The Prader-Willi syndrome: A study of 40 patients and a review of the literature. *Medicine, 62,* 59–80.

Carr, W., Moe, J., Winter, R., & Lonstein, J. (1980). Treatment of idiopathic scoliosis in the Milwaukee Brace. *Journal of Bone and Joint Surgery, 62,* 31–38.

Cassidy, S. (1984). Prader-Willi syndrome. *Current Problems in Pediatrics, 14,* 1–55.

Flickenger, E., Pories, W., Meelheim, H., Sinar, D., Blose, I., & Thomas, F. (1984). The Greenville gastric bypass: Progress report at three years. *Annals of Surgery, 199,* 555–562.

Fonkalsrud, E., & Bray, G. (1981). Vagotomy for treatment of obesity in childhood due to Prader-Willi syndrome. *Journal of Pediatric Surgery, 16,* 888–889.

Garty, B., Shuper, A., Mimouni, M., Varsano, I., & Kauli, R. (1982). Primary gonadal failure and precocious adrenarche in a boy with Prader-Labhart-Willi syndrome. *European Journal of Pediatrics, 139,* 201–203.

Grosfeld, J., Cocney, D. Csicsko, J., & Madvra, J. (1976). Adverse effects of jejunoileal bypass on growth and development. *Surgery, 80,* 201–207.

Gurd, A., & Thompson, T. (1981). Scoliosis in Prader-Willi syndrome. *Journal of Pediatric Orthopedics, 1,* 317–320.

Hall, B., & Smith, D. (1972). Prader-Willi syndrome: A resume of 32 cases including an instance of affected first cousins, one of whom is of normal stature and intelligence. *Journal of Pediatrics, 81,* 286–293.

Hamilton, C., Scully, R., & Kliman, B. (1972). Hypogonadotropinism in Prader-Willi syndrome. *American Journal of Medicine, 52,* 322–329.

Hartford, C. (1984). Near total gastric bypass for morbid obesity. *Archives of Surgery, 119,* 282–286.

Holm, V. (1981). Medical management of Prader-Willi syndrome. In V. Holm, S. Sulzbacher, & P. Pipes (Eds.), *Prader-Willi syndrome*. (pp. 261–268). Baltimore: University Park Press.

Holm, V., & Laurnen, E. (1981). Prader-Willi syndrome and scoliosis. *Developmental Medicine and Child Neurology, 23,* 192–201.

Kuldau, J., & Rand, C. (1980). Negative psychiatric sequelae to jejunoileal bypass are often not correlated with operative results. *American Journal of Clinical Nutrition, 33,* 502–503.

Laurance, B., Brito, A., & Wilkinson, J. (1981). Prader-Willi syndrome after age 15 years. *Archives of Disease in Childhood, 56,* 59–80.

Laurnen, E. (1981). Scoliosis in Prader-Willi syndrome. In V. Holm, S. Sulzbacher, & P. Pipes (Eds.), *Prader-Willi syndrome*. (pp. 293–298). Baltimore: University: Park Press.

Mason, E. (1982). Vertical banded gastroplasty. *Archives of Surgery, 117,* 701–706.

McGuffin, W., & Rogol, A. (1975). Response to LH-RH and clomiphene citrate in two women with the Prader-Labhart-Willi syndrome. *Journal of Endocrinology and Metabolism, 41,* 325–331.

Nelson, R., Huse, D., Holman, R., Kimbrough, B., Wahner, H., Callaway, C., & Hayles, A. (1981). Nutrition, metabolism, body composition, and response to the ketogenic diet in Prader-Willi syndrome. In V. Holm, S. Sulzbacher, and P. Pipes (Eds.), *Prader-Willi syndrome*. (pp. 105–120). Baltimore: University Park Press.

Orenstein, D., Boat, T., Owens, R., Horowitz, J., Primiano, F., Germann, K., & Doershuk, C. (1980). The obesity hypoventilation syndrome in children with the Prader-Willi syndrome: A possible role for familial decreased response in carbon dioxide. *Journal of Pediatrics, 97,* 765–767.

Organ, C., Cegielski, M., Grabner, B., Keig, H., & Saporta, J. (1980). Jejunoileal bypass: Long-term results. *Annals of Surgery, 192,* 38–43.

Palmer, S. K. & Atlee J. L. III, (1976). Anesthesic management of the Prader-Willi syndrome. *Anesthesiology, 44,* 161–162.

Pipes, P. (1981). Nutritional management of children with Prader-Willi syndrome. In V. Holm, S. Sulzbacher, & P. Pipes (Eds.), *Prader-Willi syndrome*. (pp. 91–41). Baltimore: University Park Press.

Randolph, J., Weintraub, W., & Rigg, A. (1974). Jejunoileal bypass for morbid obesity in adolescents. *Journal of Pediatric Surgery, 9,* 341–345.

Rochester, D., & Enson, Y. (1974). Current concepts in the pathogenesis of the obesity-hypoventilation syndrome: Mechanical and circulatory factors. *American Journal of Medicine, 57,* 402–420.

Rucker, R., Horstmann, J., Schneider, P., Varco, R., & Buchwald, H. (1982). Comparisons between jejunoileal and gastric bypass operations for morbid obesity. *Surgery, 92,* 241–249.

Scott, H. (1980). Surgical experience with jejunoileal bypass for morbid obesity. *Surgical Clinics of North America, 59,* 1033–1041.

Smith, L. (1981). Modification of the gastric partitioning operation for morbid obesity. *American Journal of Surgery, 142,* 725–730.

Smith, L., Fricke, F., & Graney, A. (1983). Results and complications of gastric partitioning: Four year follow-up of 300 morbidly obese patients. *American Journal of Surgery, 146,* 815–819.

Soper, R., Mason, E., Printen, K., & Zellweger, H. (1981). Surgical treatment of morbid obesity in Prader-Willi syndrome. In V. Holm, S. Sulzbacher, & P. Pipes (Eds.), *Prader-Willi syndrome.* (pp. 121–136). Baltimore: University Park Press.

Uehling, D. (1980). Cryptorchidism in the Prader-Willi syndrome. *Journal of Urology, 124,* 103–104.

Wannarachue, N., Ruvalcaba, R., & Kelly, V. (1975). Hypogonadism in Prader-Willi syndrome. *American Journal of Mental Deficiency, 79,* 592–603.

White, J., Cheek, D., & Haller, J. (1974). Small bowel bypass is applicable for adolescents with morbid obesity. *American Surgeon, 112,* 799–806.

Yamashita, M., Koishi, K., Yamaya, R., Tsubo, T., Matube, A., & Oyama, T. (1983). Anesthetic considerations in the Prader-Willi syndrome: Report of four cases. *Canadian Anesthetic Society Journal, 30,* 179–184.

Zellweger, H., & Schneider, H. (1968). Syndrome of hypotonia-hypomentia-hypogonadism-obesity (HHHO) or Prader-Willi syndrome. *American Journal of the Diseases of Children, 130,* 588–598.

7
Parent Concerns

RONALD L. TAYLOR and MARY LOU CALDWELL

This chapter was written to provide physicians and other direct-care professionals with information regarding parent concerns and questions about Prader-Willi syndrome. At the same time, the information can be used by parents for additional insight into their unique situation. It is hoped that the information presented will result in clearer communication between parents and physicians.

Information for this chapter was gathered both informally through innumerable conversations with parents of children with Prader-Willi syndrome, and formally from the results of a questionnaire (see Appendix). The questionnaire required a considerable amount of time and effort to complete, and was sent to a limited number of parents who agreed to participate. The 12 families who were chosen represented a diverse group with different experiences. For example, some parents learned the diagnosis of Prader-Willi syndrome early in their child's life, while others waited years to find out. For some families the child with Prader-Willi syndrome was their youngest, while in others he/she was the middle or oldest sibling.

We do not suggest that this is a scientific or empirical method of collecting and reporting data. It is, however, the most appropriate method for gathering the type of information we want to report. We were simply interested in finding out parents' subjective reactions to and interpretations of a variety of situations related to having a child with Prader-Willi syndrome. Since these are only examples of parents' reactions, we have chosen to present *trends* in the responses rather than individual comments.

As the needs of individuals with Prader-Willi syndrome change, so do the concerns of their parents. For this reason, the parents' concerns will be presented in chronological fashion. Specifically, four separate time periods will be discussed: the time of their child's birth, the time from birth until they became concerned about their child's weight gain, the time from weight gain until adolescence, and the adolescent and postadolescent years. Issues such as available medical information, impact on the family, available educational/vocational programs, and specific informational needs will be addressed.

Concerns at the Time of the Birth of the Child

MEDICAL INFORMATION RECEIVED

Until recently, the diagnosis of Prader-Willi syndrome at birth was extremely rare. Until the infant started to demonstrate the phenotypic characteristics, he/she was either misdiagnosed or not diagnosed at all. Typically, the diagnoses given were related to aspects or characteristics of the syndrome (e.g., hypotonia), and the infant was treated symptomatically. In other situations, no specific diagnosis was given but rather a general indication of the specific problems was noted. These included characteristics such as breathing or crying problems and poor suck reflex. In several instances, the parents were told that their child was retarded or that it was suspected that he/she might be.

When parents were asked about the prognosis given for their child, three types of responses emerged. One group indicated that their child was given a poor prognosis with a high probability of having significant cognitive limitations. Another group indicated that no prognosis was given (implicitly because the diagnosis was not known). The last group mentioned prognostic information that is specifically related to Prader-Willi syndrome (e.g., eventual obesity). More than likely, this information was given at a later time during their child's life since no diagnosis was given at birth. This point indicates the need for parents to keep good records regarding the developmental/medical history of their child. On several occasions, contradictory statements were made by parents. For example, they would state that no diagnosis was given during this time period, but would mention prognostic information related to the syndrome itself.

The birth of a child can be a trying and anxious time under the best of conditions. The feelings are multiplied when it is documented or at least suspected that the child is in some way "handicapped." Both the type of information given as well as the manner in which it is presented can have long-term effects on the parents' behavior and attitude toward their child. Parents had mixed reactions about the manner in which medical information was explained to them. Many stated that the physician used understandable language and showed a genuine concern. Others stated that the physician was not helpful at all. Most agreed that the amount of information given to them was insufficient.

IMPACT ON THE FAMILY

Approximately half of the parents participating in our survey indicated that the birth of their child had no effect on their marital relationship. The remaining parents were in disagreement as to the effect; about half indicated that it strengthened the relationship as a result of mutual support, while the other half indicated that it caused marital problems. From this pattern of reactions, it seems that the inclusion of a child with Prader-Willi syndrome in the family has no predictable effect on the marital relationship. The effect seems to be very specific to the individual family situation.

When asked if the birth of the child caused any problems with siblings, the response pattern was very similar. In other words, about half indicated that there was no effect, while the other half was split in its response. Some felt that the children in the family were drawn closer together while others felt that the children felt frustration and embarrassment.

About half of the parents indicated that there was undue pressure from family members (e.g., grandparents of the child). These respondents indicated that the family members did not understand the situation and tried to impose there own child-rearing philosophies/suggestions. The other half indicated that there was no pressure from family members.

It appears from the pattern of parent reactions that the effect of a birth of a child with Prader-Willi syndrome on family dynamics is situation-specific. In other words, there appears to be no clear-cut trend, either positive or negative, that would allow any prediction as to the effect on the family. Perhaps more investigation, or at least acknowledgement of the family dynamics prior to the birth of the child might result in better predictions.

INFORMATIONAL NEEDS

At the time of the birth of their child, many parents wanted diagnostic information and respite care. Most individuals indicated that they needed information about how to deal with the child's unique problems, and emotional support to help them cope with the pressures. When asked about their greatest concern at the time their child was born, the majority of parents indicated that it was uncertainty about the future, and how they would be able to take care of a handicapped child with special needs.

The majority of parents indicated that the best information they received about their child came from their pediatrician or other physician. Several indicated that they turned to hospitals, medical schools, and clinics for information. Many parents, however, indicated that they did not receive satisfactory information when there child was born. Interestingly, the vast majority of parents indicated that of all the information they have now about their child, the one thing that they wished that they had had at birth was the diagnosis of, and prognosis for, their child. Perhaps giving the parents at least a "range of prognosis" might provide them with a clearer understanding of what might happen in the future.

Concerns from the Time of the Birth of The Child to the Onset of Weight Gain

MEDICAL INFORMATION RECEIVED

The age of their child at which the parents started to show concern about weight gain varied tremendously. Some parents indicated that they started becoming concerned when their child was 6 months old, while other parents indicated that they did not become concerned until age of 7 years. The majority of the parents, however, said that they became concerned when their child was approximately 2 to 3 years old.

During this time period, a few of the parents indicated that their child was diagnosed as having Prader-Willi syndrome. The vast majority, however, indicated that no diagnosis (or a characteristic-specific diagnosis such as hypotonia) was given. Again, very little prognostic information was given to the parents, except for those whose children were diagnosed as having Prader-Willi syndrome. These parents were given a somewhat bleak picture of the future of their child, including mental retardation, inevitable obesity, and central nervous system dysfunction.

The majority of parents indicated that during this time period the physician was helpful and understandable, although even for those parents whose children had been diagnosed, little information was available about the syndrome.

IMPACT ON THE FAMILY

In contrast to the time of the birth of their child, the parents indicated that their was no marital tension during this time period. Some parents indicated that they felt sorrow at this time, while others felt guilt and helplessness regarding the child's weight gain. Similarly, none of the parents indicated that there was any sibling problems (other than that usually expected). Also, most indicated that there was little interference from outside family members, although a few parents indicated that family had unrealistic hopes that the child's problem would "go away" or that he/she would outgrow the problems.

INFORMATIONAL NEEDS

When asked what resources or services they needed at this time, many still indicated that they primarily wanted a correct diagnosis. Other needs indicated were programs or techniques of weight management. Also, many parents mentioned respite care and support from other parents.

The Time from Weight Gain to the Beginning of Adolescence

One of the reported characteristics of Prader-Willi syndrome is the lack of secondary sex characteristics. As such, the period of adolescence is sometimes difficult to identify or define for this population. Of the parents questioned, about half indicated that they were uncertain of the age at which their child entered adolescence. Others indicated that they were told by their endocrinologist that their child entered adolescence between about 12 to 15 years of age. A relatively small percentage of the parents indicated that their children did display typical physical signs of adolescence (facial and/or pubic hair) at about 13 to 14 years of age. One parent indicated that her child demonstrated appropriate social adolescent. behavior such as interest in the opposite sex. A very small percentage of the parents indicated that they knew their child had entered adolescence when they started to exhibit stubbornness, temper tantrums, and other behaviors traditionally associated with Prader-Willi syndrome during this time period.

MEDICAL INFORMATION RECEIVED

The majority of parents indicated that the diagnosis of Prader-Willi syndrome was made during this time period (mostly between the ages of 3 and 10). A small percentage of parents indicated that the diagnosis of Prader-Willi syndrome was not made but that the endocrinologist noted metabolic problems and hormone deficiencies. Of those parents whose children were diagnosed during this time, the prognostic information varied significantly. Some physicians told the parents that their child would be retarded and overweight, no matter what was done. Others indicated that the child would not necessarily be retarded, and that the weight could be controlled. One physician simply listed the reported characteristics, but noted that each case was individual. It seems very important that parents receive information noting that the characteristics among individuals with Prader-Willi syndrome do vary. First, if parents know that variation exists, they are less likely to doubt the diagnosis if the exact pattern of characteristics are not met. Secondly, they will be less likely to set up a self-fulfilling prophecy (e.g., all individuals with this syndrome have temper tantrums, my child has this syndrome, therefore my child will have temper tantrums). Those whose children were diagnosed as having endocrinological problems were given a good prognosis, assuming that appropriate hormone therapy was utilized. The majority of parents indicated that information given to them during this time was both helpful and understandable. Several admitted, however, that the information was incomplete and that little was known about their child's syndrome.

IMPACT ON THE FAMILY

About half of the parents indicated that there was no marital problem during this time period. The other half noted that there were varying degrees of tension, primarily related to the issue of diet and weight control techniques. The majority of parents indicated, however, that there was not a problem among the siblings other than the usual type encountered during this time period. Similarly, the majority indicated that there was no undue pressure by outside family members at this time. However, about half indicated that they started having problems with their child's relationship with neighbors. These problems consisted of temper tantrums, stealing, and being called names.

INFORMATIONAL NEEDS

As the child entered the school-age years, the resources and other needs requested by the parents changed somewhat. Although there was still a general need for respite care and support, there was also an indication for counseling, physical therapy, speech therapy, tutoring, and appropriate special education programs. Similarly, the parents felt that the best information that they received during this time came not only from physicians but also from school personnel. Many also indicated that information from the Prader-Willi Syndrome Association (PWSA) and various University programs focusing on the syndrome was quite helpful. When asked what their greatest concern was during this time, the majority noted behavior problems and weight control. Many also expressed concern about the future (i.e., what will happen to their child when they are too old to take care of or control their child).

EDUCATIONAL EXPERIENCES OF THE CHILD

As mentioned previously, the children's educational experiences started during this time period. When asked about these experiences the parents gave a variety of responses. The majority indicated that the child was receiving some type of special education program for behavior disordered, learning disabled, or mildly (educable) retarded students. Several felt that the school-based program in special education was very appropriate and a positive experience for their child. Others indicated that the school experience was negative and that their child was constantly in trouble because of temper tantrums, stubbornness, and stealing. It appeared that the children's attitude and behavior were related to their specific educational program and/or teacher and that no generalizations regarding their school behavior at this age should be made.

Adolescence and Postadolescence

The adolescent years represent a unique set of circumstances and situations for the parents of individuals with Prader-Willi syndrome. In addition to the usual pressures felt during this time, several other concerns were voiced including financial considerations as well as decisions regarding future living arrangement for their children.

MEDICAL INFORMATION RECEIVED

Although a significant number of children had received diagnoses prior to the adolescent years, several parents indicated that it was not until their child was approximately 15 to 17 years old that a diagnosis of Prader-Willi syndrome was made. Of those parents who indicated that their child was diagnosed during this time, almost all noted that the information regarding prognosis and the future was not very helpful. Again, some parents mentioned that the physician simply listed the characteristics of the syndrome, while others noted that the physician emphasized the limitations of their child and the need for residential or institutional placement.

IMPACT ON THE FAMILY

Interestingly, the majority of parents noted that during this time period there was marital discord primarily related to depression, tension, and the uncertainty of the future of their child. Others noted, however, that once the diagnosis was made there was a feeling of relief. There also seemed to be a significant amount of sibling problems during this time period. These problems ranged from jealousy (by the individual with Prader-Will syndrome of his sibling) to extreme overprotection of the individual with the syndrome by the sibling. In other situations there was the expression of fear and misunderstanding. Overall, there was little mention of any problems with outside family members during this time, although about half noted that there were continuing problems with neighbors (primarily related to temper tantrums and food stealing).

INFORMATIONAL NEEDS

The resources that the parents needed or wished that they had had during this period changed drastically from previous time periods. The need for financial information such as social security insurance was evident. There was also a trend indicating their need for information regarding future living arrangements for their child. The usual, consistent expression for the need for respite care and educational services was mentioned. When asked what their greatest concern was at this time, the parents consistently mentioned three: (1) the child's welfare and future (including future living arrangements); (2) financial security; (3) weight and behavioral control. Most of the parents noted that they wished that they had had information regarding effective diet control and knowledge of various sources of financial reimbursement during that time period.

Unlike previous years in which the physician was mentioned as being the best source of information to the parents, there was little mention of the physician during this time. Most of the parents noted that they got their best information through reading, parent groups, the PWSA, and various University-based programs (most notably Florida Atlantic University and the University of Washington).

EDUCATIONAL EXPERIENCES OF THE CHILD

There was a tremendous amount of difference in the types of educational programs that the children were receiving at this time. Some were receiving prevocational or vocational training at settings such as habilitation centers or sheltered workshops. Others continued in their various public school placements. Overall, it seemed that the educational placement was related to individual needs, as well as strengths and limitations, and not to Prader-Willi syndrome per se.

LIVING ARRANGEMENTS FOR THEIR CHILD

The last set of questions related to the living arrangement the parents wanted for their child. The majority of parents indicated that their child was still living at home, although a few mentioned residential schools and group homes. Almost unanimously, the parents voiced the need for group homes for their children. The majority also noted that the group home should be limited only to those individuals with Prader-Willi syndrome.

Conclusions: Suggestions for Physicians and Parents

MEDICAL INFORMATION RECEIVED

Parents consistently stated that they valued the medical information they received and wished that they had had more. Overall, the majority of parents felt that their physician gave them information in a relatively straightforward and understandable manner. The most valuable piece of medical information seemed to be the diagnostic label. Many parents felt relief and understanding when the diagnosis was finally given to them. Conversely, several felt anguish, tension, and guilt prior to receiving the diagnosis because they did not have a "reason" to explain their child's problem. With more information becoming available about Prader-Willi syndrome, more physicians should become aware and able to make a diagnosis earlier in a child's life.

Another important issue involves telling parents about the range of characteristics associated with Prader-Willi syndrome and that not every child will have all of these characteristics. As more research is conducted and many of these characteristics are challenged (e.g., see Chapter 3, this volume), this information becomes even more important.

Several of the chapters in this volume have provided information suggesting that the prognosis of Prader-Willi syndrome needs to be amended somewhat. In other words, information regarding weight control (the child will inevitably gain weight, the child will be unable to lose weight) needs to be placed within an appropriate context. These and other reported characteristics should not be thought of as an inevitable result of the syndrome. Parents need to be told that through careful planning, and a lot of hard work, the future of their children does not have to be as bleak as was once suggested. In a certain sense, the diagnosis of Prader-Willi syndrome becomes a double-edged sword. On one hand, it gives relief to the parents, yet on the other hand might lead them into accepting the "inevitable" manifestations of the syndrome. Clearly, the physician has a very important role in explaining all this information to parents.

One final note should be made regarding medical information. We noted that several parents were unsure about the time at which their child reached certain developmental milestones (this is certainly not an uncommon occurence among parents in general). It is, however, important that parents be encouraged to keep good records regarding their child's development and medical information given to them throughout the years. Understandably, with all the uncertainty about their child's future this does not appear at that time to be an important issue. It could, however, provide important information at a later date.

IMPACT ON THE FAMILY

It appears that there were certain time periods during which the child with Prader-Willi syndrome had the greatest impact on the family. One time was at the birth of the child while the other was when the child reached adolescence. At these times there seemed to be more marital tension and problems with siblings than at any other period. Certainly, one could build a strong case for these two time periods being difficult for any parent, much less those parents of a handicapped child.

Overall, there appeared to be no universal effect on the family of having a child with Prader-Willi syndrome. It seemed to magnify whatever family dynamics were already in place.

INFORMATIONAL NEEDS

It was clear that parents turned to their physicians for the majority of their informational needs, particularly during the first few years of their child's life. Most notably, the parents were seeking a medical diagnosis that would explain their child's problems. In fact, until a diagnosis was made, this seemed to be the *primary* concern of the parents. In addition, there was considerable concern for prognostic information. Even after the diagnosis was made, parents wanted to know what to expect about their child's future. A related concern was the issue of living arrangements, particularly after their child was older. Information related to group homes, etc., should be made available to parents.

Not surprisingly, most parents wanted and requested information related to sources of financial support (e.g., social security insurance). Physicians should be aware of the various available resources to help allay the parents' financial burden and/or provide the names of community-based resources (e.g., United Way, Association for Retarded Citizens) that could give them support and information.

Other concerns related to the need for more information about the syndrome and the availability of a support group. Physicians should be aware fo the PWSA, an organization that acts as a clearinghouse for information. The PWSA is a national parent support group that was founded in 1975. In addition to a national conference every year, there is also a bimonthly newsletter that disseminates a large volume of lay literature about the syndrome. In addition, there are local chapters that offer parents the opportunity to meet and discuss common concerns and problems. The address of the PWSA is: Prader-Willi Syndrome Association, 5515 Malibu Drive, Edina, Minnesota, 55436.

Appendix

Appendix

Parent Questionnaire

The following questions relate to the time at which your child was born:

1. Was any diagnosis given at this time? If so, what? If not, did you suspect that your child had any type of problem?

2. If a diagnosis was given at this time, what information was given to you regarding expected progress, prediction of future, etc.?

3. Did the physician explain things to you in an understandable fashion, or did he/she use technical and unfamiliar terms? Explain if you wish.

4. At that time, did the situation create any tension between you and your spouse? Explain if you wish.

5. At that time, did the situation create difficulties with other children in the household? Explain if you wish.

6. What types of special resources did you need at that time?

7. Were there any undue pressures from family members (e.g., grand-parents, aunts, uncles) related to the situation? Explain if you wish.

8. What was your greatest concern at that time?

9. Where did you get your best information regarding your child/ situation?

10. What do you know now that you would like to have known then?

The following questions relate to the time from the birth of your child until you became concerned about your child's weight gain:

1. At what age did your child's weight gain start to concern you?

2. Was any diagnosis given during that time? If so, what? Who gave it?

3. If a diagnosis was given during that time, what information was given to you regarding expected progress, prediction of future, etc.?

4. Did the physician (or other individual) explain things to you in an understandable fashion, or did he/she use technical and unfamiliar terms? Explain if you wish.

5. During that time, did the situation create any tension between you and your spouse? Explain if you wish.

6. During that time, did the situation create difficulties with other children in the household? Explain if you wish.

7. What types of special resources did you need during that time?

8. Were there any undue pressures from family members (e.g., grandparents, aunts, uncles) related to the situation? Explain if you wish.

9. What was your greatest concern during that time?

10. Where did you get your best information regarding your child/situation?

11. What do you know now that you would like to have known then?

These questions relate to the time from when you were concerned about weight gain until your child entered adolescence.

1. How did you determine that your child had entered adolescence? At what age did this occur?

2. Was any diagnosis given during that time? If so, what? Who gave it?

3. If a diagnosis was given during that time, what information was given to you regarding expected progress, prediction of future, etc.?

4. Did the physician (or other individual) explain things to you in an understandable fashion, or did he/she use technical and unfamiliar terms? Explain if you wish.

5. During that time, did the situation create any tension between you and your spouse? Explain if you wish.

6. During that time, did the situation create difficulties with other children in the household? Explain if you wish.

7. What types of special resources did you need during that time?

8. Were there any undue pressures from family members (e.g., grandparents, aunts, uncles) related to the situation? Explain if you wish.

9. What was your greatest concern during that time?

10. Where did you get your best information regarding your child/situation?

11. What do you know not that you would like to have known then?

12. Did you or your child have any interactions/problems with neighbors that you feel were a result of Prader-Willi syndrome?

13. Describe your child's school experiences during this time.

These questions relate to the postadolescent years.

1. Was any diagnosis given during that time? If so, what? Who gave it?

2. If a diagnosis was given during that time, what information was given to you regarding expected progress, prediction of future, etc.?

3. Did the physician (or other individual) explain things to you in an understandable fashion, or did he/she use technical and unfamiliar terms? Explain if you wish.

4. During that time, did the situation create any tension between you and your spouse? Explain if you wish.

5. During that time, did the situation create difficulties with other children in the household? Explain if you wish.

6. What types of special resources did you need during that time?

7. Were there any undue pressures from family members (e.g., grandparents, aunts, uncles) related to the situation? Explain if you wish.

8. What was your greatest concern during that time?

9. Where did you get your best information regarding your child/ situation?

10. What do you know now that you would like to have known then?

11. Did you or your child have any interactions/problems with neighbors that you feel were a result of Prader-Willi syndrome?

12. Describe your child's school and postschool experiences during that time.

13. What living situations are available to your child?

14. What living situations would you like available for your child?

15. What vocational/career training, information, etc., has your child received? Who gave it?

Thank You Very Much

Author Index

Subject Index